Wound Care

made

Incredibly

Visual!™

Wolters Kluwer | Lippincott Williams & Wilkins
Health

Philadelphia · Baltimore · New York · London
Buenos Aires · Hong Kong · Sydney · Tokyo

Staff

Executive Publisher
Judith A. Schilling McCann, RN, MSN

Editorial Director
David Moreau

Clinical Director
Joan M. Robinson, RN, MSN

Art Director
Mary Ludwicki

Senior Managing Editor
Jaime Stockslager Buss, MSPH, ELS

Clinical Project Manager
Carol A. Saunderson, RN, BA, BS

Editor
Gale Thompson

Clinical Editor
Jana L. Sciarra, RN, MSN, CRNP

Copy Editors
Kimberly Bilotta (supervisor), Scotti Cohn, Amy Furman, Shana Harrington, Dorothy P. Terry, Pamela Wingrod

Designer
Lynn Foulk

Illustrators
Esteban Cabrera, Judy Newhouse, Bot Roda, Betty Winnberg

Photographer
Wendy L. Rhodes

Digital Composition Services
Diane Paluba (manager), Joyce Rossi Biletz

Associate Manufacturing Manager
Beth J. Welsh

Editorial Assistants
Megan L. Aldinger, Karen J. Kirk, Jeri O'Shea, Linda K. Ruhf

Design Assistant
Georg W. Purvis IV

Indexer
Barbara Hodgson

WCIV010507

Library of Congress Cataloging-in-Publication Data

Wound care made incredibly visual.
  p. ; cm. — (Incredibly visual)
  Includes bibliographical references and index.
  1. Wounds and injuries — Nursing — Handbooks, manuals, etc. 2. Wounds and injuries — Nursing — Atlases. I. Lippincott Williams & Wilkins. II. Series.
  [DNLM: 1. Wounds and Injuries — nursing — Atlases. 2. Wounds and Injuries — nursing — Handbooks. WY 49 W938 2008]
  RD93.95.W69 2008
  617.1 — dc22
  ISBN-13: 978-1-58255-554-6 (alk. paper)
  ISBN-10: 1-58255-554-0 (alk. paper) 2007005867

Contents

The Year's Best Dressed

EXCESS Hollywood

My favorite part of any awards show is the parade down the red carpet, where the stars always dress to the nines. And this year's *Wound Care Made Incredibly Visual* Awards were no different.

From Al Ginate to Hydro Colloid, all of the stunning wound care stars were there to celebrate the importance of proper wound care in managing patient health.

Janice M. Beitz, RN, PhD, CS, CNOR, CWOCN
Associate Professor of Nursing
LaSalle University School of Nursing & Health Sciences
Philadelphia

Monica Beshara, RN, CWOCN, MS, NP-C
Program Director
Wound Healing & Hyperbaric Medicine Center
Saint Joseph's Hospital of Atlanta
Atlanta, Ga.

Carol Calianno, RN, MSN, CWOCN
Wound, Ostomy, Continence Nurse Specialist
Jeanes Hospital—Temple Health System
Philadelphia

Tracy A. Robinson, RN, BSN, CWOCN
Wound, Ostomy, Continence Nurse
MacNeal Hospital
Berwyn, Ill.

Tracey Siegel, RN, MSN, CWOCN, APN
Nursing Instructor
Charles E. Gregory School of Nursing
Perth Amboy, N.J.

Patricia A. Slachta, PhD, APRN, BC, CWOCN
Nursing Faculty
Division of Health Sciences
Technical College of the Low Country
Beaufort, S.C.

Cynthia A. Worley, CWOCN
Wound, Ostomy, Continence Nurse
University of Texas M.D. Anderson Cancer Center
Houston

Karen Zulkowski, DNS, RN, CWS
Associate Professor
Montana State University—Bozeman
Billings

1
Skin anatomy and physiology

Beauty may be only skin deep, but in my line of work, that's important!

Anatomy

The skin, or integumentary system, is the largest organ in the body. It accounts for about 6 to 8 lb (2.5 to 3.5 kg) of a person's body weight and has a surface area of more than 20 square feet. The living cells in the skin receive oxygen and nutrients through an extensive network of small blood vessels.

Collaboration is key. Skin is made up of separate layers that function as a single unit.

Cross section of the skin

Stratum corneum

Stratum granulosum

Stratum spinosum

Stratum basale

Dermal papillae

Pore of sweat gland

Krause's end-bulb

Free nerve ending

Meissner's corpuscle

Sebaceous gland

Arrector pilli muscle

Ruffini's corpuscle

Collagen fiber

Hair bulb

Eccrine sweat gland

Sensory nerve fibers

Autonomic nerve fibers

Epidermis

Dermis

Subcutaneous tissue (hypodermis)

Artery

Vein

> Hair and sweat glands help stabilize the skin's structural networks.

Functions of the skin layers

Layer	Description
Epidermis	▪ Outermost layer ▪ Consists of five sublayers ▪ Formed mainly by keratinocytes (cells that are continuously generated and migrate from the underlying dermis and die upon reaching the surface) ▪ Contains melanocytes (give skin and hair their color), Langerhans cells (provide the skin with immunological function), and Merkel cells (serve as markers of tactile function; confined to the lips and fingertips) ▪ Regenerates itself every 4 to 6 weeks ▪ Serves as a protective layer against water loss and physical damage
Dermis	▪ Composed of collagen fibers (give skin its strength), elastin fibers (provide elasticity), and an extracellular matrix (contributes to skin's strength and pliability) ▪ Consists of two sublayers: the papillary dermis (outer layer composed of collagen and reticular fibers) and the reticular dermis (inner layer formed by thick networks of collagen bundles that anchor onto subcutaneous tissue and underlying support structures) ▪ Contains blood and lymphatic vessels (supply nutrition and remove wastes), nerve fibers, hair follicles, sebaceous and sweat glands, and fibroblast cells (important in the production of collagen and elastin) ▪ Supplies nutrition to the skin and supports the skin's structure and strength
Subcutaneous tissue (hypodermis)	▪ Subdermal layer of adipose and connective tissue ▪ Contains major blood vessels, lymph vessels, and nerves ▪ Insulates the body, absorbs shocks to the skeletal system, and helps skin move easily over underlying structures

A closer look at epidermal layers

The epidermis consists of five distinct layers. The innermost layer contains protrusions (called *rete pegs* or *epidermal ridges*) that extend down into the dermis. Surrounded by vascularized dermal papillae, these protrusions support the epidermis and facilitate the exchange of fluids and cells between skin layers.

> Let me get this straight: the skin has three main layers. Of those three layers, the outermost layer has five layers of its own. If that were a cake, I'd need a lot of icing.

Dead keratinocytes

Stratum corneum

Stratum lucidum

Stratum granulosum

Stratum spinosum

Stratum germinativum

Basement membrane

Papillary dermis

Keratinocyte   Langerhans cell   Melanocyte   Merkel cell

The stratum corneum (a superficial layer of dead skin cells) has contact with the environment. The cells here shed daily and are replaced with cells from the layer beneath it.

The stratum lucidum (a single layer of cells) is most evident in areas where skin is thick—such as the soles—and appears to be absent where skin is especially thin—such as the eyelids.

The stratum granulosum (one to five cells thick) aids keratin formation.

The stratum spinosum is where cells begin to flatten as they migrate toward the skin surface.

The stratum germinativum, or stratum basale, is one cell thick and is the only layer in which cells undergo mitosis to form new cells.

Blood supply

The skin receives its blood supply through vessels that originate in the underlying muscle. Here, arteries branch into smaller vessels, which then branch into the network of capillaries that permeate the dermis and subcutaneous tissue.

Only capillaries have walls thin enough to let solutes pass through. These thin walls allow nutrients and oxygen to pass from the bloodstream into the interstitial space around skin cells. At the same time, waste products pass into the capillaries and are carried away.

Epidermis

Terminal arteriole

Capillary

Postcapillary venule

Papillary dermis

Upper superficial venular plexus

Superficial arterial plexus

Deep superficial venular plexus

Reticular dermis

Descending venule

Ascending arteriole

Elastic fibers

Subcutaneous tissue

Physiology

Skin performs, or participates in, a host of vital functions. Damage to skin impairs its ability to carry out these important functions.

Functions of the skin

Function		Description
	Protection	■ Acts as a physical barrier to microorganisms and foreign matter, protecting the body against infection ■ Protects underlying tissue and structures from mechanical injury ■ Prevents the loss of water, electrolytes, proteins, and other substances
	Sensory perception	■ Contains nerve endings ■ Allows for perception of pain, pressure, heat, and cold to identify potential dangers and avoid injury
	Thermoregulation	■ Contains nerves, blood vessels, and eccrine glands in the dermis to control body temperature ■ Causes blood vessels to constrict (reducing blood flow and conserving heat) when exposed to cold or internal body temperature falls ■ Causes small arteries in the skin to dilate and increases sweat production to promote cooling when skin becomes hot or internal body temperature rises
	Excretion	■ Transmits trace amounts of water and body wastes to the environment ■ Allows the skin to maintain thermoregulation and electrolyte and hydration balances ■ Prevents dehydration by ensuring that the body doesn't lose too much water
	Metabolism	■ Helps to maintain the mineralization of bones and teeth ■ Synthesizes vitamin D (which is crucial to the metabolism of calcium and phosphate) when exposed to the ultraviolet spectrum in sunlight
	Absorption	■ Allows for the absorption of some drugs directly into the bloodstream

As people age, their skin's ability to sense pressure, heat, and cold becomes impaired, even though the number of nerve endings in the skin remains unchanged.

Aging and skin function

With aging, the skin undergoes a number of changes that increase the risk of wound development and impair the ability of wounds to heal.

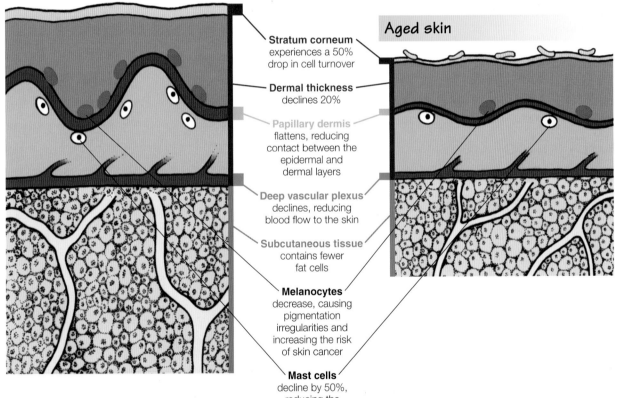

Youthful skin

Aged skin

Stratum corneum experiences a 50% drop in cell turnover

Dermal thickness declines 20%

Papillary dermis flattens, reducing contact between the epidermal and dermal layers

Deep vascular plexus declines, reducing blood flow to the skin

Subcutaneous tissue contains fewer fat cells

Melanocytes decrease, causing pigmentation irregularities and increasing the risk of skin cancer

Mast cells decline by 50%, reducing the inflammatory response

Able to label?

Identify the five layers of the epidermis indicated on this illustration.

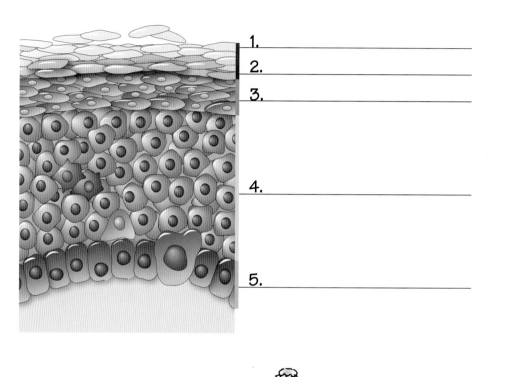

1. _____

2. _____

3. _____

4. _____

5. _____

Rebus riddle

Sound out each group of pictures and symbols to reveal an important fact about the skin.

the ~~skin~~ is ↑ of

3 🦁 🍰 ⬇

Answers: Able to label? 1. Stratum corneum, 2. stratum lucidum, 3. Stratum granulo-sum, 4. Stratum spinosum, 5. Stratum germinativum; Rebus riddle The skin is made up of three main layers.

2 Wound healing

Trust me... sometimes things don't knit back together just like you'd like them to.

Types of wound healing

Any break in the skin is considered a wound. The extent and type of damage—as well as other intrinsic factors, such as patient circulation, nutrition, and hydration—influence the rate of wound repair. Wounds can heal, or close, through primary intention, secondary intention, or tertiary intention.

Primary intention

Wounds that heal through primary intention usually don't involve the loss of tissue. Examples include surgical wounds, superficial traumatic wounds, and first-degree sunburn.

Clean incision	Early suture	Hairline scar

> Wounds that heal by primary intention get it right the first time.

Wound has well-approximated edges.

Clean edges can be pulled together neatly.

Because there's no loss of tissue and little risk of infection, these wounds usually heal in 4 to 14 days and result in minimal scarring.

Wounds that heal by secondary intention need a second chance to get it right. Luckily, granulation tissue can "fill in" the gap.

Secondary intention

A wound that involves some degree of tissue loss heals by secondary intention. Pressure ulcers, burns, dehisced surgical wounds, and traumatic injuries are examples of this type of wound. These wounds take longer to heal, result in scarring, and have a higher rate of complications than wounds that heal by primary intention.

Gaping irregular wound	Granulation	Epithelium growth over scar

Edges can't be easily approximated.

Wound fills with granulation tissue.

A scar forms and reepithelialization occurs, primarily from the wound edges.

Tertiary intention

Wounds are sometimes left open for several days to allow edema or infection to resolve or for exudate to drain. These wounds heal by tertiary intention, also known as *delayed primary closure*. After the problem resolves, these wounds are closed with sutures or some other type of skin closure. Wounds that first require debridement also heal by tertiary intention.

Open wound	Increased granulation	Late suturing with wide scar

Wound is intentionally kept open (typically for 3 to 5 days) to allow edema or infection to resolve or to permit removal of exudate.

Wound fills with granulation tissue.

Wound is sutured late and a wide scar results.

Wounds that heal by tertiary intention need three steps: draining, "filling" by granulation, and then suturing.

Phases of wound healing

The healing process is the same for all wounds, whether the cause is mechanical, chemical, or thermal. Health care professionals discuss the process of wound healing in four specific phases: hemostasis, inflammation, proliferation, and maturation.

Wound healing process

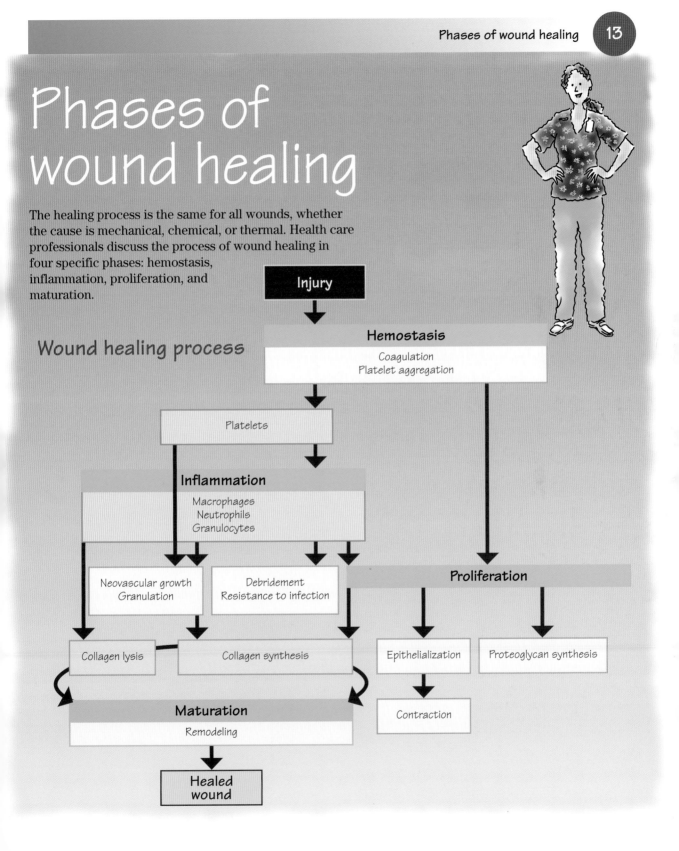

Injury

Hemostasis
Coagulation
Platelet aggregation

Platelets

Inflammation
Macrophages
Neutrophils
Granulocytes

Neovascular growth
Granulation

Debridement
Resistance to infection

Proliferation

Collagen lysis

Collagen synthesis

Epithelialization

Proteoglycan synthesis

Maturation
Remodeling

Contraction

Healed
wound

Hemostasis

When tissue is damaged, serotonin, histamine, prostaglandins, and blood from the injured vessels fill the area. Blood platelets form a clot, and fibrin in the clot binds the wound edges together.

Inflammation

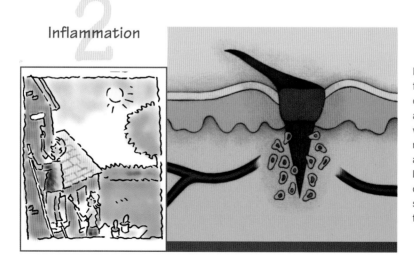

Lymphocytes initiate the inflammatory response, increasing capillary permeability. Wound edges swell; white blood cells from surrounding vessels move in and ingest bacteria and cellular debris, demolishing the clot. Redness, warmth, swelling, pain, and loss of function may occur.

Proliferation

Adjacent healthy tissue supplies blood, nutrients, fibroblasts, proteins, and other building materials needed to form soft, pink, and highly vascular granulation tissue, which begins to bridge the area.

Maturation

Fibroblasts in the granulation tissue secrete collagen, a gluelike substance. Collagen fibers crisscross the area, forming scar tissue. Meanwhile, epithelial cells at the wound edge multiply and migrate toward the wound center. A new layer of surface cells replaces the layer that was destroyed. New, healthy tissue or granulation tissue (if the blood supply is inadequate) appears.

Just as movies don't always reflect real life, healing rarely occurs in this strict order. Typically, the phases of wound healing overlap.

Damaged tissue (including lymphatics, blood vessels, and stromal matrices) regenerates. Collagen fibers shorten, and the scar diminishes in size. Scar size may decrease and normal function return or the scar may hypertrophy, leading to the formation of a keloid and the development of contractures.

Recognizing wound failure to heal

Sign	Causes	Interventions
Wound bed		
Too dry	■ Exposure of tissue and cells normally in a moist environment to air ■ Inadequate hydration	■ Add moisture regularly. ■ Use a dressing that maintains moisture, such as a hydrocolloid or hydrogel dressing.
No change in size or depth for 2 weeks	■ Pressure or trauma to the area ■ Poor nutrition, poor circulation, or inadequate hydration ■ Poor control of disease processes such as diabetes ■ Inadequate pain control ■ Infection	■ Reassess the patient for local or systemic problems that impair wound healing, and intervene as necessary.
Increase in size or depth	■ Debridement ■ Ischemia due to excess pressure or poor circulation ■ Infection	■ If caused by debridement, no intervention is necessary. ■ Poor circulation may not be resolvable, but consider adding warmth to the area and administering a vasodilator or antiplatelet medication. ■ If caused by infection, administer topical or systemic antimicrobials, as ordered.
Necrosis	■ Ischemia	■ Perform debridement if the remaining living tissue has adequate circulation.
Increase in drainage or change in drainage from clear to purulent	■ Autolytic or enzymatic debridement ■ Infection	■ If caused by autolytic or enzymatic debridement, no intervention is necessary; an increase or change of color in drainage is expected because of the breakdown of dead tissue. ■ If debridement isn't the cause, assess the wound for infection. ■ If caused by infection, administer topical or systemic antimicrobials, as ordered.
Tunneling	■ Pressure over bony prominences ■ Presence of foreign body ■ Deep infection	■ Protect the area from pressure. ■ Irrigate and inspect the tunnel as carefully as possible for a hidden suture or leftover bit of dressing material. ■ If the tunnel doesn't shorten in length each week, thoroughly clean and obtain a tissue biopsy for infection and, with a chronic wound, for possible malignancy.

Sometimes, no matter what you do, a plot just fails to come together.

Sign	Causes	Interventions
Wound edges		
Red, hot skin; tenderness; and induration	▪ Inflammation due to excess pressure or infection	▪ Protect the area from pressure. ▪ If pressure relief doesn't resolve the inflammation within 24 hours, topical antimicrobial therapy may be indicated.
Maceration (white skin)	▪ Excess moisture	▪ Protect the skin with petrolatum ointment or a barrier wipe. ▪ If practical, obtain an order for a more absorptive dressing.
Rolled skin edges	▪ Too-dry wound bed	▪ Obtain an order for moisture-retentive dressings. ▪ If rolling isn't resolved in 1 week, debridement of the edges may be necessary.
Undermining or ecchymosis of surrounding skin (loose or bruised skin edges)	▪ Excess shearing force to the area	▪ Initiate measures to protect the area, especially during patient transfers.

Effects of aging on wound healing

Skin changes that occur with aging cause healing time to be prolonged in elderly patients.

Factors that delay healing

■ Slower turnover rate in epidermal cells
■ Poor oxygenation of the wound (due to increasingly fragile capillaries and a reduction in skin vascularization)
■ Impaired function of the respiratory or immune system
■ Reduced dermal and subcutaneous mass (leading to an increased risk of chronic pressure ulcers)
■ Lack of tensile strength in healed wounds, making them prone to reinjury

Factors that complicate healing

■ Poor nutrition and hydration
■ Presence of a chronic condition
■ Use of multiple medications

Physical changes from aging—such as a declining sense of smell and taste and decreased stomach motility—can affect a patient's nutritional and fluid intake.

Other factors can also affect our nutritional status, such as loose dentures, financial concerns, or problems preparing or obtaining food.

Complications of wound healing

Dehiscence and evisceration may require emergency surgery, especially when an abdominal wound is involved. If a wound opens without evisceration, it may need to heal by secondary intention.

Wound dehiscence

Dehiscence is a separation of skin and tissue layers. It's most likely to occur 3 to 11 days after the injury was sustained and may follow surgery.

Evisceration of bowel loop

Evisceration is similar to dehiscence but involves protrusion of underlying visceral organs as well.

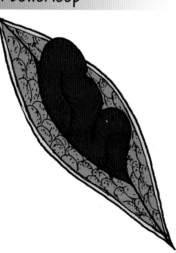

Poor nutrition and advanced age increase a patient's risk of dehiscence and evisceration.

Detecting wound dehiscence

Signs of dehiscence include an abscess or a gush of serosanguineous fluid from the wound. The patient may also report a "popping" sensation at the wound site.

Dehisced abdominal wound (with a colostomy)

Dehisced healing abdominal incision

Colostomy

Red granulation tissue

Yellow fibrin slough

take note

Documenting wound dehiscence and evisceration

| 08/24/06 | 0945 | During dressing change at 0925, noted dehiscence of distal 2" of midline abdominal incision. Superficial layers of tissue observed; no evisceration noted. Pt. placed in reclined position with knees flexed. Pt. states, "I felt something give when I coughed." Wound covered with sterile 4" X 4" gauze soaked in NSS and then covered with dry sterile dressing. P 100, BP 150/84, RR 18, T 98.6° F. Dr. McBride notified at 0930. Adhesive strips ordered and applied to wound. Pt. to be kept on bed rest until Dr. McBride visits pt. at 1030. Pt. instructed to stay in bed with knees flexed and to call nurse for assistance with moving in bed. Reviewed splinting incision with pillow if he has to cough or sneeze. Call bell placed within reach, and pt. demonstrated how to use it. ————————————— *Maureen Dunlop, RN* |

Infection

Infection is a relatively common complication of wound healing that should be addressed promptly.

Infection can lead to a cellulitis or bacterial infection that spreads to surrounding tissue. So, be alert!

Signs of infection

- ■ Redness and warmth of the margins and tissue around the wound
- ■ Fever
- ■ Edema
- ■ Pain (or a sudden increase in pain)
- ■ Pus
- ■ Increase in exudate or a change in its color
- ■ Odor
- ■ Discoloration of granulation tissue
- ■ Further wound breakdown or lack of progress toward healing

Recognizing wound infection

Clean wound

The wound here is healing properly. It's clean and has no redness, swelling, or drainage.

Infected wounds

These wounds show signs of infection.

Redness and swelling along incision line and in surrounding tissue

Redness

Pus

Fistulas and sinus tracts

A fistula is an abnormal passage between an organ or a vessel and another organ, vessel, or area of the skin. A sinus tract, also known as *tunneling*, is a channel that extends through part of a wound and into adjacent tissue. These complications can result in dead space and infection.

This tunnel covers a lot of territory underground. Likewise, sinus tracts are wound channels that can extend into subcutaneous tissue and muscle.

Undermining

Undermining is tissue destruction that occurs around a wound's edges, causing the skin to come away from the base of the wound (even though it may appear intact). It can develop into sinus tracts to nearby tissue.

Undermining should be carefully probed to determine how far it extends under intact skin.

Undermining is tissue destruction around the borders of a wound. It results in a wound bed that extends under the skin.

Matchmaker

Match each illustration to the proper phase of wound healing.

A. _____

B. _____

C. _____

D. _____

1. Hemostasis
2. Inflammation
3. Proliferation
4. Maturation

My word!

Unscramble the names of four complications of wound healing. Then use the circled letters to answer the question posed.

Question: Which sign of failure to heal is caused by ischemia and requires wound debridement?

1. icravesitone __ _ ⃝ _ _ _ _ ⃝ _ _ _ _ _ _
2. sciencehed _ ⃝ _ _ ⃝ _ _ ⃝ _ _
3. niceifnot _ _ _ _ _ ⃝ _ _ ⃝ _
4. usaflit _ _ ⃝ _ _ _ _

Answer: _ _ _ _ _ _ _ _ _

3
Wound assessment

Assess my wounds? How, pray tell, can mere words describe the depth of my despair?

Wound classification

The words used to describe a wound must communicate the same thing to members of the health care team, insurance companies, regulators, the patient's family and, ultimately, the patient himself. The best way to classify wounds is to use the basic system described here, which focuses on three categories of fundamental characteristics:

> Even when the wound bed appears healthy, red, and moist, if healing fails to progress, consider the wound to be chronic.

1 Wound age

2 Wound depth

3 Wound color

Wound age

The first step in classifying a wound is to determine whether the wound is acute or chronic. Be careful, you can't base your determination solely on time because no set time frame specifies when an acute wound becomes chronic.

Characteristics of acute and chronic wounds

Acute	Chronic
■ New or relatively new wound	■ May develop over time
■ Occurs suddenly	■ Healing has slowed or stopped
■ Healing progresses in a timely, predictable manner	■ Typically heals by secondary intention
■ Typically heals by primary intention	■ Examples: Pressure, vascular, and diabetic ulcers
■ Examples: Surgical and traumatic wounds	

Wound depth

Wound depth can be classified as partial thickness or full thickness.

> In the case of pressure ulcers, wound depth allows you to stage the ulcer according to the classification system developed by the National Pressure Ulcer Advisory Panel. (See chapter 6, Pressure ulcers.)

Partial-thickness wound

Partial-thickness wounds involve only the epidermis or extend into the dermis but not through it.

Full-thickness wound

Full-thickness wounds extend through the dermis into tissues beneath and may expose adipose tissue, muscle, or bone.

Measuring wound depth

To measure the depth of a wound, you'll need gloves, a cotton-tipped swab, and a disposable measuring device. This method can also be used to measure wound tunneling or undermining.

1 Put on gloves and gently insert the swab into the deepest portion of the wound.

2 Grasp the swab with your fingers at the point that corresponds to the wound's margin. You can carefully mark the swab where it meets the edge of the skin.

3 Remove the swab and measure the distance from your fingers or from the mark on the swab to the end of the swab to determine the depth.

Wound color

The Red-Yellow-Black Classification System is a commonly used approach that can help you determine how well a wound is healing and develop effective wound care management plans.

Red wounds

Red indicates normal healing. When a wound begins to heal, a layer of pale pink granulation tissue covers the wound bed. As this layer thickens, it becomes beefy red.

RED WOUNDS = HEALING

Granulation tissue in an abdominal wound

Granulation tissue base in a diabetic foot ulcer

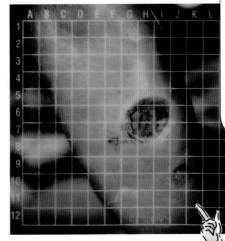

The grid in this photo allows for measuring wound area (the squares are counted and multiplied) and monitoring wound progress (the number of squares should decrease as healing progresses).

Yellow wounds

Fibrin left over from the healing process usually appears as yellow slough or dead tissue on the wound base. This slough, or soft necrotic tissue, provides a medium for bacterial growth.

Sacral pressure ulcer with 75% of the surface area covered in yellow necrotic slough

Diabetic foot ulcer with a slough-covered base and calloused edges

Black wounds

Black, the least healthy wound color, signals necrosis. Dead avascular tissue (known as *eschar*) slows healing and provides a site for microorganisms to proliferate.

Black pressure ulcer

Black ischemic toe ulcers

When eschar covers a wound, accurate assessment of wound depth is difficult and should be deferred until eschar is removed.

Best dressed

Tailoring wound care to wound color

Wound color	Management technique
Red	■ Cover the wound, keep it moist and clean, and protect it from trauma. ■ Use a transparent dressing (such as Tegaderm or OpSite) over a gauze dressing moistened with normal saline solution, or use a hydrogel, foam, or hydrocolloid dressing to insulate and protect the wound.
Yellow	■ Clean the wound and remove the yellow layer. ■ Cover the wound with a moisture-retentive dressing (such as a hydrogel or foam dressing or a moist gauze dressing with or without a debriding enzyme). ■ Consider hydrotherapy with whirlpool or pulsatile lavage.
Black	■ Debride the wound as ordered. Use an enzyme product (such as Accuzyme or Panafil), conservative sharp debridement, or hydrotherapy with whirlpool or pulsatile lavage. ■ For wounds with inadequate blood supply and uninfected heel ulcers, don't debride. Keep them clean and dry.

Classifying multicolored wounds

If you note two or even all three colors in a wound, classify the wound according to the least healthy color present. For example, if your patient's wound appears both red and yellow, classify it as a yellow wound.

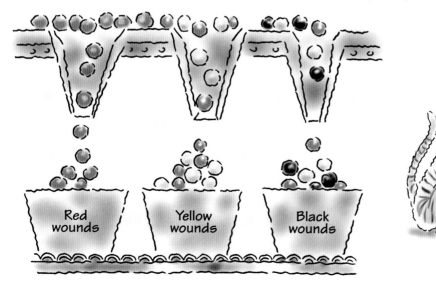

Yes, I know you're mostly yellow, but for classification purposes, we're going to have to call you black.

Wound terminology

Every wound has a different size, shape, and color, which can make accurate documentation challenging. However, understanding and using standard terminology can make the job easier.

Call 'em like you see 'em

When you visually examine a wound, look for the following key characteristics.

What do you see?

Beefy red, bumpy, shiny tissue in the base of an ulcer

- This indicates **granulation tissue**.
- As a wound heals, it develops more and more granulation tissue.

Pale or dark pink skin

- This indicates **epithelial tissue**.
- Epithelial tissue first appears at ulcer borders in full-thickness wounds and as islands around hair follicles in partial-thickness wounds.

Moist yellow or gray area of tissue that's separating from viable tissue

- This is **slough** and indicates soft, necrotic tissue.
- Slough provides an ideal medium for bacterial growth.

Thick, hard, leathery black tissue

- This is **eschar** and indicates dry, necrotic tissue.
- For healing to occur, necrotic tissue, drainage, and metabolic wastes must be removed.

Waterlogged skin; possibly white at the wound edges

- This indicates **macerated tissue**.
- A dressing that provides too much moisture can cause maceration of surrounding skin, unless the skin is protected.
- Other common causes of maceration include wound drainage or contamination with urine or feces.

Wound drainage

A thorough wound assessment includes assessing drainage. To begin collecting information about wound drainage, inspect the dressing as it's removed and record your findings.

Drainage descriptors

Description	Color and consistency
Serous	▪ Clear or light yellow ▪ Thin and watery
Sanguineous	▪ Red (with fresh blood) ▪ Thin
Serosanguineous	▪ Pink to light red ▪ Thin ▪ Watery
Purulent	▪ Creamy yellow, green, white, or tan ▪ Thick and opaque

take note

Documenting wound drainage

| 11/30/06 | 1330 | Dressing on abdominal surgical site changed. Pt. medicated with 2 mg of morphine sulfate at 1315 for comfort. Outside of dressing was dry with no obvious drainage. No oozing from edges of dressing noted at this time. Dressing removed using adhesive remover. Moderate amount of serosanguineous drainage present on interior of dressing. No odor from drainage noted. Patient tolerated procedure well. ——Leah Noble, R.N. |

Wound measurement

When measuring a wound, you must determine its length, width, and depth. (Measuring wound depth is described on page 26.) You must also measure the surrounding areas.

Length

- First, determine the longest distance across the open area of the wound—regardless of orientation.
- In this photo, note the line used to illustrate length.

Width

- Next, determine the longest distance across the wound at a right angle to the length.
- In this photo, note the relationship between length and width.

Surrounding areas

- Note areas of reddened, intact skin; indurated (or hard) skin; and white (macerated) skin.
- These areas are measured and recorded as surrounding erythema, induration, and maceration, not as part of the wound itself.

Measuring wound tunneling

Tunneling, also known as *undermining*, is tissue destruction that occurs around the wound perimeter underlying intact skin, causing the wound edges to pull away from the wound's base. Because tunneling may be more extensive in one part of a wound than another, measuring and documenting the location and depth of tunneling is an essential component of a wound assessment.

Probing the issue

■ Put on sterile gloves. Gently probe the wound bed and edges with your finger or a sterile cotton-tipped applicator to assess for wound tunneling.
■ Gently insert the applicator into the wound in the direction where the deepest tunneling occurs, as shown below.

Marking progress

■ Grasp the applicator where it meets the wound edge.
■ Remove the applicator, keeping your hand in place, and place it next to the measuring guide to determine the length of tunneling in centimeters, as shown below.

Wound documentation

Proper documentation accurately portrays the characteristics of a wound and its status in the healing process.

Think of your words as your palette, using them to paint a vivid description of your patient's wound.

memory board

Use the mnemonic device **WOUNDD PICTURE** to help you recall and organize all of the key facts that should be included in your documentation of a wound:

Wound or ulcer location

Odor (in room or just when wound is uncovered)

Ulcer category, stage (for pressure ulcer) or classification (for diabetic ulcer), and depth (partial thickness or full thickness)

Necrotic tissue

Dimension (shape, length, width, and depth)

Drainage color, consistency, and amount (scant, moderate, or large)

Pain (when it occurs, what relieves it, patient's description, and patient's rating on scale of 0 to 10)

Induration (hard or soft surrounding tissue)

Color of wound bed (red, yellow, black, or combination)

Tunneling (length and direction—toward the patient's right, left, head, or feet)

Undermining (record length and direction, using clock references to describe)

Redness or other discoloration in surrounding skin

Edge of skin loose or tightly adhered and flat or rolled under

What's missing from this picture?

Wound photography may be a routine part of your facility's wound documentation system. Photographs can provide benchmarks for and facilitate documentation of wound healing.

Even though a picture may be "worth a thousand words," remember that your assessment skills and personal observations are still essential because many wound characteristics can't be recorded accurately— or at all—on film. For example, look at the photograph below and consider which wound characteristics you can't assess. Examples include:

- location
- depth
- tunnel measurement
- odor
- feel of surrounding tissue
- pain.

All of this information is needed if the health care team is to make sound treatment decisions.

VISION QUEST

Matchmaker

Match each photo with the terminology that describes the characteristics of the wound.

1. _____   2. _____

3. _____   4. _____

A. Macerated tissue
B. Granulation tissue
C. Eschar
D. Slough

Show and tell

Describe the three steps used to measure wound depth that are shown here.

1. _____
_____
_____

2. _____
_____
_____

3. _____
_____
_____

Answers: Matchmaker 1. B, 2. C, 3. A, 4. D; Show and tell 1. Insert the swab into the deepest portion of the wound. 2. Grasp the swab at the point where it meets the wound's margin. 3. Remove the swab and measure the distance from your finger to the end of the swab.

4
Wound care procedures

Listen up, people! We have a lot of procedures to cover before we can "wrap things up."

DIRECTOR

Cleaning a wound

The goal of wound cleaning is to remove debris and contaminants from the wound without damaging healthy tissue. After an initial cleaning, wounds should be cleaned as needed and before a new dressing is applied.

Step by step

As you follow these steps, be sure to observe standard precautions. Follow facility protocols regarding use of clean or sterile technique.

1 **Remove the soiled dressing.** Roll or lift an edge of the dressing and then gently remove it while supporting the surrounding skin. When possible, remove the dressing in the direction of hair growth.

2 **Inspect the dressing and wound.** Note the color, amount, and odor of drainage and necrotic debris.

When cleaning a wound, move from the least contaminated area to the most contaminated area. Also, be sure to use a clean gauze pad for each wipe.

Cleaning techniques

To clean a linear shaped wound (such as an incision), gently wipe from top to bottom in one motion, starting directly over the wound and moving outward, as shown below.

For an open wound (such as a pressure ulcer), gently wipe in concentric circles, starting directly over the wound and moving outward, as shown below.

3 **Clean the wound.** Moisten gauze pads either by dipping the pads in wound cleaning solution and wringing out excess or by using a spray gun bottle to apply solution to the gauze.

4 Dry the wound. Using the same procedure as for cleaning a wound, dry the wound using dry gauze pads.

5 Reassess the condition of the skin and wound. Note the character of the clean wound bed and surrounding skin.

Wound reassessment algorithm

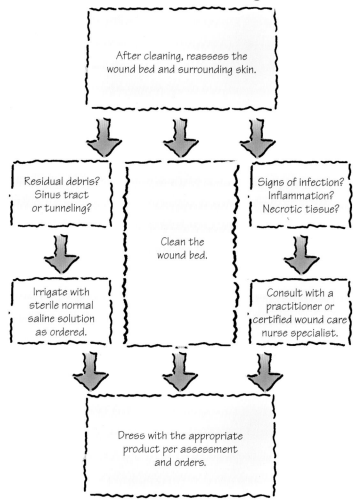

After cleaning, reassess the wound bed and surrounding skin.

Residual debris? Sinus tract or tunneling?

Clean the wound bed.

Signs of infection? Inflammation? Necrotic tissue?

Irrigate with sterile normal saline solution as ordered.

Consult with a practitioner or certified wound care nurse specialist.

Dress with the appropriate product per assessment and orders.

6 Pack or dress the wound as ordered.

Choosing a cleaning agent

The type of cleaning agent you'll use on a wound depends on the wound type and characteristics.

- Most commonly used cleaning agent
- Provides a moist environment
- Promotes granulation tissue formation
- Causes minimal fluid shifts in healthy adults

- Sometimes used to clean infected or newly contaminated wounds
- May damage healthy tissue and delay wound healing

> Watch for patient sensitivity to povidone-iodine.

Types of antiseptic solutions

Hydrogen peroxide
- Used to clean or irrigate as mechanical debridement aid
- Promotes vasodilation through warmth of foaming action
- Reduces inflammation
- Commonly used half-strength
- Avoid use in sinus tracts due to risk of air embolism

Acetic acid
- Used to treat *Pseudomonas* infection
- Verify active infection by culture before use
- 0.5% to 5% strength depending on order

Sodium hypochlorite (Dakin's solution)
- Used to kill gram-negative bacteria per culture
- Slightly dissolves necrotic tissue
- Must be freshly prepared every 24 hours (solution is unstable)

Povidone-iodine
- Used to kill broad spectrum of bacteria
- May dry and stain the surrounding skin; protect from contact
- Toxic with prolonged use or over large areas
- Avoid use in patients with thyroid disease

Chlorhexidine
- Used to kill gram-positive and gram-negative bacteria
- Must be diluted

Irrigating a wound

Irrigation serves to:
- clean tissues
- flush cell debris and drainage from an open wound
- prevent premature surface healing over an abscess pocket or infected tract.

Normal saline solution is the optimal irrigant because it won't disrupt healthy tissue or wound-healing cells.

Step by step

As you follow these steps, be sure to observe standard precautions and maintain sterile technique.

1 **Prepare the solution and equipment.** Fill the irrigating device with irrigating solution.

2 **Irrigate the entire wound thoroughly.**
Gently instill a slow, steady stream of solution into the wound (below left). Make sure the solution flows from the clean area to the dirty area of the wound to prevent contamination of clean tissue. To prevent tissue damage, don't force the needle or angiocatheter into the wound. Irrigate until you've administered the prescribed amount of solution or until the solution returns clear. Note the amount of solution administered. Keep the patient positioned to allow complete wound drainage (below right).

Devices used to irrigate a wound should provide gentle, low-pressure irrigation and may include a bulb syringe or a 35-ml piston syringe with an 18-gauge needle or angiocatheter.

3 **Clean and dry the skin.** Use normal saline solution on the periwound skin, and then pat it dry with gauze.

4 **Pack or dress the wound as ordered.**

Packing a wound

Packing is used for mechanical debridement of a wound and to prevent surface healing before deep healing. The type of packing material used depends on the size of the wound and the amount of exudate.

> Times have changed! Cotton mesh gauze used to be the standard in packing material. Today, you have more options.

Step by step

As you follow these steps, be sure to observe standard precautions.

1 **Make sure the packing material is moist.** Use a slight amount of sterile normal saline solution if needed.

2 **Pack the wound.** Use sterile forceps and cotton-tipped applicators as needed.
- Fluff the moist sterile packing pad or strip to unclump it.
- Loosely but thoroughly pack the wound. Note that packing the wound too tightly can create pressure damage on the granulating cells.
- Cover all the wound surfaces and edges.
- Pack only in the wound bed because packing material can macerate intact tissue.

3 **Dress with dry sterile gauze.**

Dressing a wound

I'm here at the annual Wound Dressing Competition. As any fan of this competition knows, the winning dressing always provides an optimal environment in which the body can heal.

Competition is fierce. Contestants are judged on their ability to keep wounds moist, absorb drainage, conform to the wound, and be comfortable. Let's go to the competition floor.

The composite dressing is taking his turn. He has scored a perfect 10 in his compulsories and is now performing his individual program. What a unique combination! Let's see how he thinks he scored.

I did my best in adhering to the surrounding skin, decreasing the need for a secondary dressing, and showing my user-friendly side. Let's hope the judges also find me cost-effective.

Can I tell it like it is? I think you've impressed the judges. We'll have to see how the other contestants perform, though.

Wound dressing algorithm

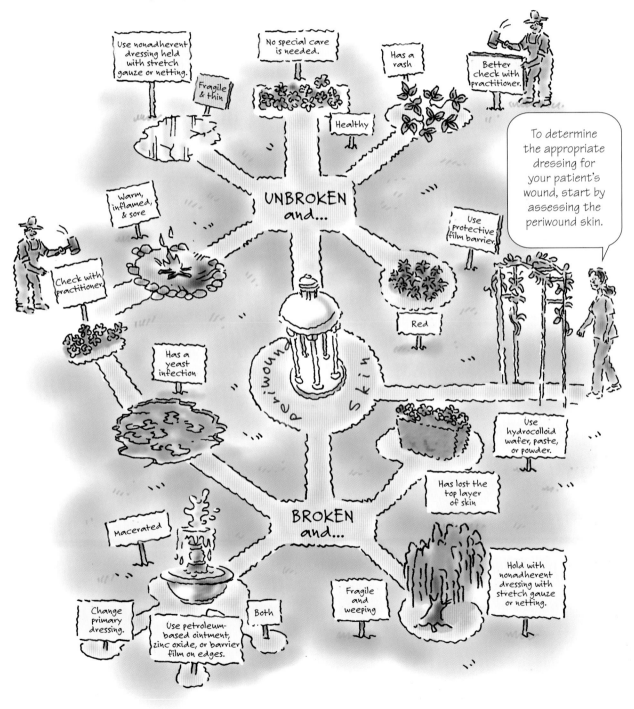

Best dressed

Step-by-step wound dressing

Regardless of the dressing or topical agent you use, follow your facility's protocol or the manufacturer's instructions for applying the wound dressing.

Type of dressing	Application method
Alginate	▪ Apply the dressing to the wound surface. ▪ Cover the area with a secondary dressing (such as gauze pads or transparent film), as ordered. ▪ Secure the dressing with tape or elastic netting. ▪ If the wound is heavily draining, change the dressing once or twice daily for the first 3 to 5 days. As drainage decreases, change the dressing less frequently—every 2 to 4 days or as ordered. When the drainage stops or the wound bed looks dry, stop using alginate dressings.
Foam	▪ Gently lay the dressing over the wound. ▪ Use tape, elastic netting, or gauze to hold the dressing in place. ▪ Change the dressing when the foam no longer absorbs exudate.
Hydrocolloid	▪ Choose a clean, dry, presized dressing or cut one to overlap the wound by about 1″ (2.5 cm). ▪ Remove the dressing from its package. ▪ Pull the release paper from the adherent side of the dressing. ▪ Apply the dressing to the wound, carefully smoothing out wrinkles and avoiding stretching the dressing. ▪ Hold the dressing in place with your hand (the warmth from your hand will mold the dressing to the skin). ▶ ▪ If the dressing's edges need to be secured with tape, apply a skin sealant to the intact skin around the wound. After the area dries, tape the dressing to the skin. The sealant protects the skin from tape burns and skin stripping and promotes tape adherence. Avoid using tension or pressure when you apply the tape. ▪ Change the dressing every 2 to 7 days as necessary; change it immediately if the patient complains of pain, the dressing no longer adheres, or leakage occurs.

Type of dressing	Application method	
Hydrogel	▪ Apply a moderate amount of gel to the wound bed. ▪ Cover the area with a secondary dressing (gauze, transparent film, or foam). ▪ Change the dressing daily or as needed to keep the wound bed moist. ▪ If the dressing you select comes in sheet form, cut the dressing to overlap the wound by 1″ (2.5 cm); then apply as you would a hydrocolloid dressing. *Note:* Hydrogel dressings also come as prepackaged, saturated gauze for wounds with cavities that require "dead space" to be filled. Follow the manufacturer's directions to apply these dressings.	
Moist saline gauze	▪ Moisten the dressing with normal saline solution. ▪ Wring out excess fluid. ▶ ▪ Gently place the dressing onto the wound surface, molding the moist gauze around the wound. ▶ ▪ To separate surfaces within the wound, gently guide the gauze between opposing wound surfaces. To avoid damage to tissues, don't pack the gauze tightly. ▪ Apply a sealant or barrier to protect the surrounding skin from moisture. ▪ Change the dressing frequently enough to keep the wound moist.	
Transparent	▪ Select a dressing to overlap the wound by 1″ to 2″ (2.5 to 5 cm). ▪ Gently lay the dressing over the wound; avoid wrinkling the dressing. To prevent shearing force, don't stretch the dressing over the wound. Press firmly on the edges of the dressing to promote adherence. ▪ Change the dressing every 3 to 5 days, depending on the amount of drainage. If the seal is no longer secure, change the dressing.	

Applying a wound pouch

A wound with copious, excoriating drainage may need to have a pouch applied. A wound pouch collects drainage and helps protect the surrounding skin.

Step by step

When applying a wound pouch, wear a gown and a face shield or mask and goggles in case the drainage splashes. Be sure to follow standard precautions when performing the following steps.

1 **Measure the wound.** Use a disposable measuring tape to obtain the wound's length and width.

2 **Cut an opening in the wafer.** The opening should be ⅜″ (1 cm) larger than the wound (as shown below).

3 **Apply a skin protectant as needed.** Note that some protectants are incorporated within the wafer and also provide adhesion.

4 Press the contoured pouch opening around the wound. Start at the lowest edge of the wound to catch any drainage (as shown below).
– Make sure the drainage port at the bottom of the pouch is closed firmly to prevent leaks.
– Be gentle but firm to avoid causing pain; offer to hold the wafer in place while the patient presses, if preferred.

5 Empty the pouch as needed. Insert the bottom half of the pouch into a graduated biohazard container, and open the drainage port (as shown below).
– Note the color, consistency, odor, and amount of fluid.
– If ordered, obtain a culture specimen and immediately send it to the laboratory.
– Wipe the bottom of the pouch and the drainage port with a gauze pad to remove drainage, which could irritate the patient's skin or cause an odor.
– Reseal the port.

6 Change the pouch as needed. Only change the pouch if it leaks or fails to adhere as more frequent changes may irritate the patient's skin.

The surface swab technique obtains bacteria colonized only on the wound's surface. For a more accurate culture, needle aspiration of fluid or punch tissue biopsy should be used.

Collecting a wound culture

Infected wounds (those with heavy bacterial or fungal overgrowth) are unable to properly heal. Cultures can help to determine the involved organism and guide treatment. One common wound culture collection method is the surface swab technique. Other methods, including syringe aspiration and punch tissue biopsy, are performed by advanced practice nurses and physicians.

Although you may not want me in the wound bed, once you find me there, be sure to transport the specimen to the collection tube carefully, so that I don't die.

Step by step

When obtaining a wound culture, follow standard precautions and maintain sterile technique throughout each of these steps.

1 **Inspect and irrigate.** After inspecting the wound, thoroughly irrigate it with sterile saline solution.

2 **Rotate a sterile swab along all areas of the wound.** Gently twist the calcium alginate or rayon swab (not cotton-tipped) on the sides and base of the wound, crossing the entire surface of the wound. To ensure all possible areas of infection have been swabbed, use the 10-point coverage system.

3 **Place the swab in the appropriate culture medium.** If the wound is open and has viable tissue, immediately place the swab in an aerobic culture tube. If the wound has necrotic tissue or sinus tracts, obtain both an aerobic and an anaerobic culture.

4 **Label the culture tube.** Immediately send it to the laboratory.

Collecting an anaerobic specimen

Because most anaerobes die when exposed to oxygen, they must be transported in tubes filled with carbon dioxide or nitrogen. Before specimen collection, the small inner tube containing the swab is held in place with a rubber stopper.

After collecting the specimen, quickly replace the swab in the inner tube and depress the plunger to separate the inner tube from the stopper. The swab is forced into the larger tube, exposing the specimen to a carbon dioxide–rich environment.

Before   After

Debriding a wound

Debridement is the removal of necrotic (dead) tissue and debris (such as eschar) from a wound. When combined with optimal nutrition, circulation, mobility, and attitude toward healing, debridement can help to promote wound healing.

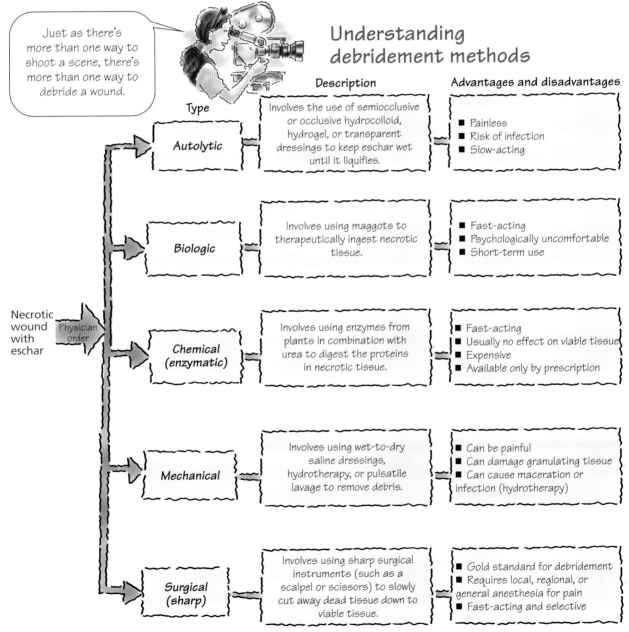

Just as there's more than one way to shoot a scene, there's more than one way to debride a wound.

Understanding debridement methods

Type	Description	Advantages and disadvantages
Autolytic	Involves the use of semiocclusive or occlusive hydrocolloid, hydrogel, or transparent dressings to keep eschar wet until it liquifies.	■ Painless ■ Risk of infection ■ Slow-acting
Biologic	Involves using maggots to therapeutically ingest necrotic tissue.	■ Fast-acting ■ Psychologically uncomfortable ■ Short-term use
Chemical (enzymatic)	Involves using enzymes from plants in combination with urea to digest the proteins in necrotic tissue.	■ Fast-acting ■ Usually no effect on viable tissue ■ Expensive ■ Available only by prescription
Mechanical	Involves using wet-to-dry saline dressings, hydrotherapy, or pulsatile lavage to remove debris.	■ Can be painful ■ Can damage granulating tissue ■ Can cause maceration or infection (hydrotherapy)
Surgical (sharp)	Involves using sharp surgical instruments (such as a scalpel or scissors) to slowly cut away dead tissue down to viable tissue.	■ Gold standard for debridement ■ Requires local, regional, or general anesthesia for pain ■ Fast-acting and selective

Necrotic wound with eschar — Physician order

Assisting in sharp debridement

Sharp debridement helps to create a blood-rich, uninfected wound surface in which granulation can occur. Advanced practice nurses with specific training in this care can remove tissue that's dead or loose (has a clearly visible line where viable tissue begins). However, only a surgeon can debride wounds that cover very large areas, are deep and very close to vital structures, or whose edges can't be readily distinguished from viable tissues. General or regional anesthesia is required for this procedure.

Nonviable tissue

Step by step

Follow standard precautions and maintain a sterile field and sterile technique when assisting with sharp debridement.

1 Administer an analgesic, as ordered. Give an oral drug 20 minutes before debridement, or an I.V. analgesic immediately before the procedure.

2 Assist the practitioner as needed. Provide assistance as the practitioner lifts the edges of eschar, holds necrotic tissue taut with sterile forceps, and cuts dead tissue from the wound. Irrigate the wound as necessary.

Healthy tissue

3 Apply pressure to bleeding tissues. If bleeding occurs, apply gentle pressure with sterile 4″ × 4″ gauze pads.

4 Treat and dress the site as ordered. Apply topical medications and replace and secure the dressing, as ordered.

In debridement, dead tissue is removed, which exposes healthy tissue and increases the size of the wound.

Documenting wound care

Documentation checklist

When documenting wound care, be sure to include:

☑ date, time, and type of wound care performed
☑ amount of soiled dressing and packing removed
☑ type, color, consistency, and amount of drainage
☑ wound appearance (size, condition of margins, presence of necrotic tissue)
☑ presence of odor
☑ presence and location of drains
☑ additional procedures, such as irrigation, packing, or application of a topical medication
☑ type and amount of new dressing or pouch applied
☑ patient's tolerance of the procedure.

Document special or detailed wound care instructions and pain management steps on the care plan. Also record the amount of drainage on the intake and output sheet.

take note

Documenting wound care

| 03/26/07 | 1430 | Dressing removed from abdominal incision. 2-cm round area of serosanguineous drainage noted on dressing. No odor noted. Incision well approximated except for 1.5-cm area at distal end of incision. Wound culture obtained and sent to lab. Incision cleaned with sterile NSS and sterile dressing applied. Pt. tolerated procedure well. ———— David Stevens, RN |

Matchmaker

Match the wound cleaning technique shown with the proper wound type for which it's used.

Show and tell

State which wound care procedure is illustrated here and explain why this method is used.

1.

2.

A. Circular wound
B. Linear wound

_____

_____

_____
_____
_____
_____
_____

5
Acute wounds

I love a script with burning passions, burning desires, and even burning buildings. But skin burns? Ouch. That's a different story entirely.

Burns

Burns are tissue injuries that result from contact with thermal, chemical, or electrical sources or from friction or exposure to the sun. They can cause cellular skin damage and a systemic response that leads to altered body function. A major burn affects every body system and organ, usually requiring painful treatment and a long period of rehabilitation.

Types of burns

First-degree

A first-degree burn causes localized injury or destruction to the skin's epidermis by direct contact (such as a chemical spill) or indirect contact (such as sunlight).

> Although a first-degree burn isn't life-threatening and doesn't disrupt the barrier function of the skin, it still hurts!

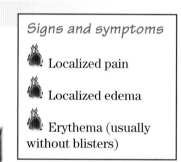

Signs and symptoms

- Localized pain
- Localized edema
- Erythema (usually without blisters)

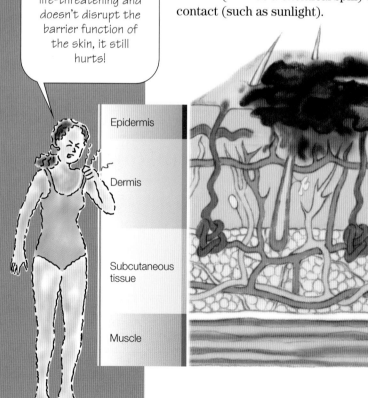

Epidermis

Dermis

Subcutaneous tissue

Muscle

Second-degree

Second-degree burns are subclassified as either **SUPERFICIAL** partial-thickness burns or **DEEP** partial-thickness burns.

Epidermis

Dermis

Subcutaneous
tissue

Muscle

This first-degree burn resulted from sunburn. Notice the localized erythema and absence of blisters characteristic of first-degree burns.

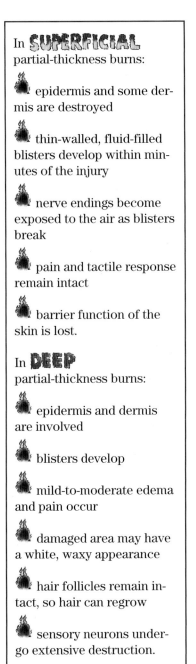

In **SUPERFICIAL** partial-thickness burns:

🔥 epidermis and some dermis are destroyed

🔥 thin-walled, fluid-filled blisters develop within minutes of the injury

🔥 nerve endings become exposed to the air as blisters break

🔥 pain and tactile response remain intact

🔥 barrier function of the skin is lost.

In **DEEP** partial-thickness burns:

🔥 epidermis and dermis are involved

🔥 blisters develop

🔥 mild-to-moderate edema and pain occur

🔥 damaged area may have a white, waxy appearance

🔥 hair follicles remain intact, so hair can regrow

🔥 sensory neurons undergo extensive destruction.

Thin-walled blisters

This photo shows a deep partial-thickness burn. Note the white, waxy appearance. In this instance, the large bullae will most likely be ruptured.

Bullae

You can easily see the dermis in this deep partial-thickness burn.

Dermis

Third-degree

Also known as *full-thickness burns*, these burns:

🔥 extend through the epidermis and dermis and into the subcutaneous tissue layer

🔥 may involve muscle, bone, and interstitial tissues

🔥 may have a white, brown, or black leathery appearance without blisters

🔥 may reveal thrombosed vessels (due to destruction of skin elasticity)

🔥 cause fluids and protein to shift from capillary to interstitial spaces within hours, causing edema

🔥 trigger an immediate immunologic response, making burn wound sepsis a potential threat.

Epidermis

Dermis

Subcutaneous tissue

Muscle

A third-degree burn results in an increased calorie demand, which increases the patient's metabolic rate.

The full-thickness burns shown in this photo resulted from being scalded in a bathtub.

The black, leathery skin and absence of blisters over this hand and wrist are characteristic of third-degree burns.

Note the thrombosed blood vessels visible in this third-degree burn of the foot.

Electrical burns

Electrical burns usually result from contact with faulty electrical wiring and cords or high-voltage power lines.

Cross-section of skin with electrical burn

Epidermis

Dermis

Subcutaneous tissue

Muscle

At the site of electrical contact, the injury may appear silver-colored, with a raised or charred area.

Tissue damage from electrical burns is difficult to assess because internal damage along the conduction pathway is commonly greater than the surface burn indicates.

The person in this photo tried to stop a fall from a ladder by grasping a high-voltage electrical line, resulting in electrocution and an electrical burn.

Estimating the extent of burns

Rule of Nines

You can quickly estimate the extent of an adult patient's burn by using the Rule of Nines. This method quantifies body surface area (BSA) in multiples of nine, giving the method its name.

To use this method, mentally assess your patient's burns according the body charts below. Add the corresponding percentages for each body section burned. Use the total—a rough estimate of the extent of the burn—to calculate initial fluid replacement needs.

> Because BSA varies with age, you'll use the Rule of Nines to estimate the extent of an adult patient's burns and the Lund-Browder classification to estimate the extent of an infant's or a child's burns.

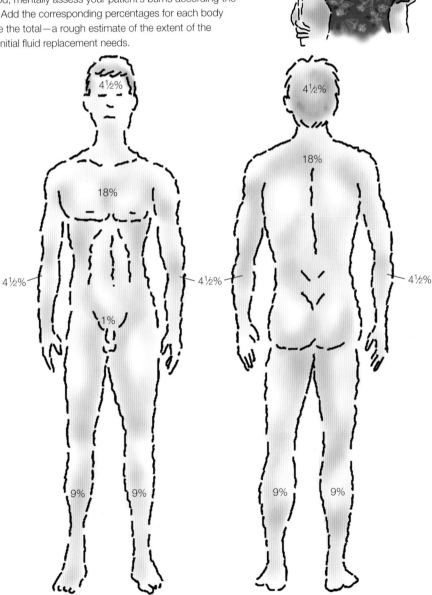

Lund-Browder classification

The Rule of Nines isn't accurate for infants or children because their body shapes, and therefore BSA, differ from those of adults. For example, an infant's head accounts for about 17% of total BSA, compared with 7% for an adult. Instead, use the Lund-Browder classification (shown below) to determine burn size for infants and children.

Percentage of burned body surface by age

	At birth	0 to 1 year	1 to 4 years	5 to 9 years	10 to 15 years	Adult
A: Half of head	9½%	8½%	6½%	5½%	4½%	3½%
B: Half of one thigh	2¾%	3¼%	4%	4¼%	4½%	4¾%
C: Half of one leg	2½%	2½%	2¼%	3%	3¼%	3½%

Biological burn dressings

Biological dressings provide a temporary protective covering for burn wounds and clean granulation tissue. They also temporarily secure fresh skin grafts and protect graft donor sites.

> In addition to stimulating new skin growth, biological dressings act like normal skin: They reduce heat loss, block infection, and minimize fluid, electrolyte, and protein losses.

Comparing biological dressings

Type	Description and uses	Nursing considerations
Cadaver (organic, homograft)	▪ Obtained at autopsy up to 24 hours after death ▪ Applied in the operating room or at the bedside to debrided, untidy wounds ▪ Available as fresh cryopreserved homografts in tissue banks nationwide ▪ Provides protection, especially to granulation tissue after escharotomy ▪ May be used in some patients as a test graft for autografting ▪ Covers excised wounds immediately	▪ Observe for exudate. ▪ Watch for signs of rejection. ▪ Keep in mind that the gauze dressing may be removed every 8 hours to observe the graft.
Pigskin (organic, heterograft or xenograft)	▪ Applied in the operating room or at the bedside ▪ Comes fresh or frozen in rolls or sheets ▪ Can cover and protect debrided, untidy wounds, mesh autografts, clean (eschar-free) partial-thickness burns, and exposed tendons	▪ Reconstitute frozen form with normal saline solution 30 minutes before use. ▪ Watch for signs of rejection. ▪ Cover with gauze dressing or leave exposed to air, as ordered.
Amniotic membrane (organic, homograft)	▪ Available from the obstetric department ▪ Must be sterile and come from an uncomplicated birth; serologic tests must be done ▪ Bacteriostatic condition doesn't require antimicrobials ▪ May be used to protect partial-thickness burns or (temporarily) granulation tissue before autografting ▪ Applied by the physician to clean wounds only	▪ Change the membrane every 48 hours. ▪ Cover the membrane with a gauze dressing or leave it exposed, as ordered. ▪ If you apply a gauze dressing, change it every 48 hours.
Biobrane (biosynthetic membrane)	▪ Comes in sterile, prepackaged sheets in various sizes and in glove form for hand burns ▪ Used to cover donor graft sites, superficial partial-thickness burns, debrided wounds awaiting autograft, and meshed autografts ▪ Provides significant pain relief ▪ Applied by the nurse	▪ Leave the membrane in place for 3 to 14 days, possibly longer. ▪ Don't use this dressing for preparing a granulation bed for subsequent autografting.

Keep in mind that a patient who has received an autograft requires care for two wounds: one at the graft site and one at the donor site.

Skin grafts

Skin grafting consists of taking healthy tissue—from either the patient (autograft) or a donor (allograft)—and applying it to an area damaged by burns, traumatic injury, or surgery.

Types of skin grafts

A burn patient may receive split-thickness grafts, full-thickness grafts, or both.

Epidermis

Dermis

Subcutaneous tissue

Muscle

Sweat gland

Hair follicle

Split-thickness skin graft

Full-thickness skin graft

Thin 0.01"

Medium 0.02"

Thick 0.035"

0.04"

Split-thickness grafts

■ Include the epidermis and part of the dermis
■ Commonly used to cover open burns
■ May be applied as a sheet (usually on the face or neck for cosmetic purposes)
■ May also be applied as a mesh (usually on extensive full-thickness burns)

Full-thickness skin grafts

■ Include the epidermis and the entire dermis
■ Contain hair follicles, sweat glands, and sebaceous glands
■ Usually used for small deep burns

Keys to a successful skin graft

✔ Clean wound granulation with adequate vascularization

✔ Complete contact of the graft with the wound bed

✔ Maintenance of sterile technique to prevent infection

✔ Adequate graft immobilization

✔ Skilled care

Common donor skin graft sites

Split-thickness graft sites

Full-thickness graft sites

Fat-dermal graft sites

Caring for a donor graft site

In autografting, tissue is removed from the patient's body using a der-matome, an instrument that cuts uniform, split-thickness skin portions (shown below). Consequently, the donor site is a partial-thickness wound, which may bleed, drain, and cause pain. Depending on the graft's thickness, tissue may be obtained from the donor site again in as few as 10 days.

Usually, a moisture vapor–permeable dressing or Xeroflo gauze is applied postoperatively to protect new epithelial proliferation.

Dressing the wound

▣ Wash your hands and put on sterile gloves.

▣ Remove the outer gauze dressings within 24 hours. Inspect the Xe-roflo gauze dressing for signs of infection; then leave it open to the air to speed drying and healing.

▣ Leave small amounts of fluid accumulation alone. Using sterile technique, aspirate larger amounts through the dressing with a small-gauge needle and syringe.

▣ Apply a lanolin-based cream daily to completely healed donor sites to keep skin tissue pliable and to remove crusts.

The donor site needs scrupulous care to prevent infection, which could cause the site to become a full-thickness wound.

Evacuating fluid from a sheet graft

When small pockets of fluid (called *blebs*) accumulate beneath a sheet graft, a physician will need to evacuate the fluid using a sterile scalpel and sterile cotton-tipped applicators. Be prepared to assist, as needed.

 The physician will carefully perforate the center of the bleb with the scalpel.

 Then he'll gently express the fluid with the cotton-tipped applicators.

! Fluid should never be expressed by rolling the bleb to the edge of the graft. This disturbs healing in other areas.

Surgical wounds

Acute surgical wounds are uncomplicated breaks in the skin that result from surgery. In an otherwise healthy individual, these types of wounds typically heal without incident.

> Never remove a surgical dressing without an order. Some dressings put pressure on the wound; others keep skin grafts intact.

Assessment

> What is this? Some type of investigation?

> Just good surgical sleuthing, sir.

First check the outside...

✔ Is the dressing stained?
  – Estimate drainage quantity.
  – Note its color, consistency, and odor.

✔ Does the patient have a drainage device?
  – Record the amount of drainage.
  – Note the color of the drainage.
  – Ensure that the device is secure and free from kinks.

✔ Does the patient have an ileostomy or colostomy?
  – Describe its output.

...then go under cover

✔ Is a healing ridge present?
  – Are there signs and symptoms of infection, such as redness, warmth, and edema along the incision line and in the surrounding area; localized pain and tenderness; fever; pus or exudate from the incision; separation of suture line?

Definition: Healing ridge

Palpable ridge that forms on each side of the wound during normal wound healing. It results from a buildup of collagen fibers, which begins to form during the inflammatory phase of wound healing and peaks during the proliferation phase (approximately 5 to 9 days postoperatively). Ridges typically fail to develop because of mechanical strain on the wound.

Warning!

Wound infection is the most common surgical wound complication and the second most common infection type that occurs during hospitalization.

Postoperative leg wound infection

> Being a good surgical sleuth means never going it alone. Train the patient to care for his wound and to monitor healing.

What to teach your patient about surgical wound care

☑ Signs and symptoms of wound infection to report immediately

☑ Procedure for taking an accurate temperature reading

☑ Proper wound care, such as keeping the incision clean and dry, proper hand-washing technique, and supplies and methods used to clean the wound

☑ Wound dressings, including the type, places to obtain them, and proper application

☑ Types and levels of permissible activity, such as lifting restrictions (if applicable), restrictions on bathing, and expectations for returning to work

☑ Follow-up appointments

Wound closure

The severity of a wound determines the type of material used to close it.

Adhesive closures

Adhesive closures, such as Steri-Strips or butterfly closures, may be used to close small wounds with scant drainage or to provide continued reinforcement after suture or staple removal.

Steri-Strips

Steri-Strips are thin strips of sterile, nonwoven tape. They're a primary means of holding a wound closed after suture removal.

Butterfly closures

Butterfly closures consist of two sterile, waterproof adhesive strips linked by a narrow, nonadhesive "bridge." They're used to hold small wounds closed to promote healing after suture removal.

I should know. Not every job calls for the same stitch.

Suture methods

Surgeons usually use sutures. If cosmetic results aren't an issue, the surgeon may choose to use skin staples or clips.

Mattress continuous suture

Connected mattress stitches with a knot at the beginning and end

Plain continuous suture

Connected stitches with the thread knotted at the beginning and end of the suture; also called a *continuous running suture*

Blanket continuous suture

Looped stitches with a knot at the beginning and end

Mattress interrupted suture

Independent stitches with both threads crossing beneath the suture line, leaving only a small portion of suture exposed on each side of the wound

Plain interrupted suture

Individual sutures sewn with a separate piece of thread; half the thread length crosses under the suture line and the other half crosses above the skin surface

Suture materials

Nonabsorbable sutures

- Used to close the skin surface
- Provide strength and immobility
- Cause minimal tissue irritation
- Consist of silk, cotton, stainless steel, or nylon

Absorbable sutures

- Used when suture removal is undesirable
- Consist of:
  - chromic catgut—a natural catgut treated with chromium trioxide to improve strength and prolong absorption time
  - plain catgut—a material that's absorbed faster and is more likely to cause irritation than chromic catgut
  - synthetic materials (such as polyglycolic acid)—materials that are replacing catgut because they're stronger, more durable, and less irritating.

Although absorbable sutures are made of a material called "catgut," I've got nothing to worry about. It's those guys whose stomachs are on the line!

Caring for and dressing surgical wounds

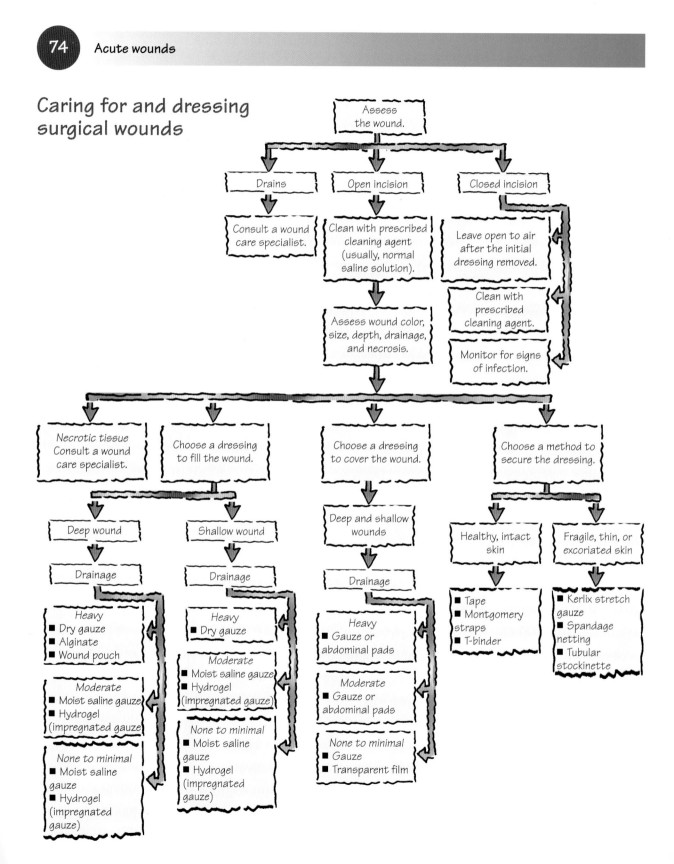

How to make Montgomery straps

An abdominal dressing requiring frequent changes can be secured with Montgomery straps to promote the patient's comfort. If ready-made straps aren't available, follow these steps to make your own:

1 Cut four to six strips of 2″ to 3″ wide hypoallergenic tape of sufficient length to allow the tape to extend about 6″ (15.2 cm) beyond the wound on each side. (The length of the tape might vary according to the patient's size and the type and amount of dressing.)

2 Fold one of each strip 2″ to 3″ (5 to 7.5 cm) back on itself (sticky sides together) to form a nonadhesive tab. Then cut a small hole in the folded tab's center, close to its top edge. Make as many pairs of straps as you'll need to snugly secure the dressing.

3 Clean the patient's skin to prevent irritation. After his skin dries, apply a skin protectant. Then apply the sticky side of each tape to a skin barrier sheet composed of opaque hydrocolloidal or nonhydrocolloidal materials, and apply the sheet directly to the skin near the dressing.

4 Thread a separate piece of gauze tie, umbilical tape, or twill tape (about 12″ [30.5 cm]) through each pair of holes in the straps, and fasten each tie as you would a shoelace. Don't stress the surrounding skin by securing the ties too tightly.

Replace Montgomery straps every 2 to 3 days or whenever they become soiled. If skin maceration occurs, place new tapes about 1″ (2.5 cm) away from irritation.

Wound care in obese patients

After surgery, obese patients experience slower wound healing because fatty tissue lacks a sufficient blood supply. Also, because excess fat strains wound edges, obese patients have an increased risk of wound dehiscence. Placing an abdominal binder (shown at left) over the surgical site will help support the incision. Specific wound care will vary according to the surgical procedure performed.

Surgical drains

Surgeons insert closed-wound drains during surgery when they expect a large amount of postoperative drainage. These drains suction serosanguineous fluid from the wound site.

  If a wound produces heavy drainage, the closed-wound drain may be left in place for longer than 1 week. Drainage must be frequently emptied and measured to maintain maximum suction and prevent strain on the suture line. Treat the tubing exit site as an additional surgical wound.

Closed-wound drainage system

A closed-wound drain consists of perforated tubing connected to a portable vacuum unit. (Hemovac and Jackson-Pratt are the most commonly used drainage systems.) The distal end of the tubing lies within the wound and usually leaves the body from a site other than the primary suture line. The drain is usually sutured to the skin. Shown below is a closed-wound drainage system in a postmastectomy patient.

To empty the drainage, remove the plug and empty it into a graduate cylinder. To reestablish suction in a Hemovac unit, compress the drainage unit against a firm surface to expel air and, while holding it down, replace the plug with your other hand (as shown above).

Follow a similar procedure to reestablish suction in a Jackson-Pratt bulb drain (shown above).

Surgical drain

Colostomy and ileostomy care

A patient with a colostomy or ileostomy wears an external pouch over the ostomy site, attached via a hydrocolloid wafer. The pouch collects fecal matter, helps control odor, and protects the stoma and peristomal skin. Most disposable pouching systems can be used for 7 days, unless a leak develops.

When selecting a pouching system, choose one that delivers the best adhesive seal and skin protection for that patient. Other considerations include the stoma's location and structure, consistency of the fecal matter, availability and cost of supplies, amount of time the patient will wear the pouch, any known adhesive allergy, and the personal preferences of the patient.

> The best time to change a pouching system is first thing in the morning or 2 to 4 hours after meals, when the bowel is least active. After a few months, most patients can predict the time that's best for them.

Transverse colostomy

Ascending colostomy

Descending colostomy

Ileostomy

Sigmoid colostomy

Comparing ostomy pouching systems

Manufactured in many shapes and sizes, ostomy pouches are fashioned for comfort, safety, and easy application. Some commonly available pouches are described here.

Disposable pouches

The patient who must empty his pouch often (because of diarrhea or a new colostomy or ileostomy) may prefer a one-piece, drainable, disposable pouch with a closure clamp attached to a skin barrier. This pouch may be used permanently or temporarily, until stoma size stabilizes.

Also disposable and made of transparent or opaque odor-proof plastic, a one-piece disposable closed-end pouch may come with a carbon filter for gas release. A patient with a regular bowel elimination pattern may choose this style for additional security and confidence.

A two-piece disposable drainable pouch with separate skin barrier permits frequent changes and also minimizes skin breakdown.

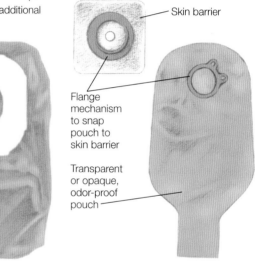

Attached adhesive seal or skin barrier

Transparent or opaque, odor-proof, plastic pouch

Bottom opening for easy drainage

Attached adhesive seal or skin barrier

Closed end to prevent leakage

Skin barrier

Flange mechanism to snap pouch to skin barrier

Transparent or opaque, odor-proof pouch

Reusable pouches

Reusable pouches come with a separate custom-made faceplate and O-ring (as shown at right). Some pouches have a pressure valve for releasing gas. The device has a 1- to 2-month life span, depending on how frequently the patient empties the pouch.

Reusable equipment may benefit a patient who needs a firm faceplate or who wishes to minimize cost. However, many reusable ostomy pouches aren't odor-proof.

Sturdy, opaque, hypoallergenic, plastic pouch

Bottom opening for easy drainage

Applying a skin barrier and pouch

Fitting a skin barrier and ostomy pouch properly can be done in a few steps. Shown here is a two-piece pouching system with flanges, which is commonly used.

1. Measure the stoma using a measuring guide.

2. Trace the appropriate circle carefully on the back of the skin barrier.

3. Cut the circular opening in the skin barrier. Bevel the edges to keep them from irritating the patient.

4. Remove the backing from the skin barrier and moisten it or apply barrier paste, as needed, along the edge of the circular opening.

5. Center the skin barrier over the stoma, adhesive side down, and gently press it to the skin.

6. Gently press the pouch opening onto the ring until it snaps into place.

Show and tell

Identify the type of burn shown in each of these photos.

1. _____

_____

2. _____

3. _____

_____

4. _____

_____

Matchmaker

Match the five suture methods shown here with their names.

1.

___

2.

___

3.

___

4.

___

5.
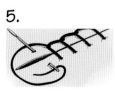
___

A. Mattress interrupted suture
B. Plain interrupted suture
C. Plain continuous suture
D. Mattress continuous suture
E. Blanket continuous suture

Answers: Able to label? 1. First-degree burn, 2. Deep partial-thickness burn, 3. Third-degree burn, 4. Second-degree burn; Matchmaker 1. D, 2. A, 3. C, 4. B, 5. E.

6 Pressure ulcers

Okay, the pressure is on. In this scene, you'll be caring for patients with pressure ulcers.

Causes

Pressure ulcers typically occur when pressure compresses soft tissue over a bony prominence. Friction and shear also contribute to the development of pressure ulcers.

Understanding the pressure gradient

A V-shaped pressure gradient results from the upward force exerted by a support surface and the downward force of a bony prominence. Pressure is greatest on tissues at the apex of the gradient and lessens to the right and left of this point.

An estimated 1 million to 1.7 million pressure ulcers occur each year in the United States, with one-half of those being stage II or greater.

Bone

Muscle

Subcutaneous fat

Dermis

Epidermis

Supporting surface

Sitting

Shoulder blade

Tailbone

Buttocks
Back of knee

Heels

Lying

Sides of feet and ankles

Front of knee

Upper thighbone

Upper hipbone

Shoulder

Side of head

These illustrations show the areas most likely to develop pressure ulcers.

Understanding shearing force

Shear is a mechanical force that occurs parallel, rather than perpendicular, to an area of tissue. In this illustration, gravity pulls the body down the incline of the bed. The skeleton and attached tissues move, but the skin remains stationary, held in place by friction between the skin and the bed linen. The skeleton and attached tissues actually slide within the skin, causing the skin to pucker in the gluteal area.

Risk factors

High-risk patients, whether in an institution or at home, should be assessed regularly for pressure ulcers. Be sure to consider all risk factors when assessing patients.

Risk factor	Considerations
Advanced age	▪ Skin becomes more fragile as epidermal turnover slows, vascularization decreases, and skin layers adhere less securely to one another. ▪ Older adults have less lean body mass and less subcutaneous tissue to cushion bony areas. ▪ Underlying problems that increase pressure ulcer risk include poor hydration and impaired respiratory and immune systems.
Immobility	▪ Immobility may be the greatest risk factor for pressure ulcer development. ▪ The patient is less able to move in response to pressure sensations and his position is changed less frequently.
Incontinence	▪ Incontinence increases a patient's exposure to moisture and, over time, increases his risk of skin breakdown. ▪ Urinary and fecal incontinence can result in excessive moisture and chemical irritation (fecal incontinence can cause more damage because of pathogens in stools).
Infection	▪ Compressed skin has a lower local resistance to bacterial infection. ▪ Infection may reduce the pressure needed to cause tissue necrosis.
Low blood pressure	▪ Low blood pressure can lead to tissue ischemia, particularly in patients with vascular disorders. ▪ As tissue perfusion drops, the skin is less tolerant of sustained external pressure, increasing the risk of damage from ischemia.
Malnutrition	▪ A strong correlation exists between poor nutrition and the development of pressure ulcers. ▪ The body requires increased protein for healing; malnutrition can lead to decreased protein levels, including decreased albumin. ▪ A direct correlation exists between pressure ulcer stage and the degree of hypoalbuminemia.

Braden Scale for Predicting Pressure Sore Risk

Tally the numbers for each description that applies to your patient. Determine your patient's risk as follows:

- 15 to 18: At risk
- 13 to 14: Moderate risk
- 10 to 12: High risk
- 9 or below: Very high risk.

Sensory perception: Ability to respond meaningfully to pressure-related discomfort

1. Completely limited	*2. Very limited*
Unresponsive (does not moan, flinch, or grasp) to painful stimuli due to diminished level of consciousness or sedation OR Limited ability to feel pain over most of body	Responds only to painful stimuli. Cannot communicate discomfort except by moaning or restlessness. OR Has a sensory impairment which limits the ability to feel pain or discomfort over ½ of body.

Moisture: Degree to which skin is exposed to moisture

1. Constantly moist	*2. Very moist*
Skin is kept moist almost constantly by perspiration, urine, etc. Dampness is detected every time patient is moved or turned.	Skin is often, but not always moist. Linen must be changed at least once a shift.

Activity: Degree of physical activity

1. Bedfast	*2. Chairfast*
Confined to bed.	Ability to walk severely limited or nonexistent. Cannot bear own weight and/or must be assisted into chair or wheelchair.

Mobility: Ability to change and control body position

1. Completely immobile	*2. Very limited*
Does not make even slight changes in body or extremity position without assistance.	Makes occasional slight changes in body or extremity position but unable to make frequent or significant changes independently.

Nutrition: <u>Usual</u> food intake pattern

1. Very poor	*2. Probably inadequate*
Never eats a complete meal. Rarely eats more than ⅓ of any food offered. Eats 2 servings or less of protein (meat or dairy products) per day. Takes fluids poorly. Does not take a liquid dietary supplement. OR Is NPO and/or maintained on clear liquids or IVs for more than 5 days.	Rarely eats a complete meal and generally eats only about ½ of any food offered. Protein intake includes only 3 servings of meat or dairy products per day. Occasionally will take a dietary supplement. OR Receives less than optimum amount of liquid diet or tube feeding.

Friction and shear

1. Problem	*2. Potential problem*
Requires moderate to maximum assistance in moving. Complete lifting without sliding against sheets is impossible. Frequently slides down in bed or chair, requiring frequent repositioning with maximum assistance. Spasticity, contractures, or agitation leads to almost constant friction.	Moves feebly or requires minimum assistance. During a move skin probably slides to some extent against sheets, chair, restraints or other devices. Maintains relatively good position in chair or bed most of the time but occasionally slides down.

Patient's name _____   Evaluator's name _____

	Date of assessment		

3. Slightly limited
Responds to verbal commands but cannot always communicate discomfort or the need to be turned.
OR
Has some sensory impairment which limits ability to feel pain or discomfort in 1 or 2 extremities.

4. No impairment
Responds to verbal commands. Has no sensory deficit which would limit ability to feel or voice pain or discomfort.

3. Occasionally moist
Skin is occasionally moist, requiring an extra linen change approximately once a day.

4. Rarely moist
Skin is usually dry; linen only requires changing only at routine intervals.

3. Walks occasionally
Walks occasionally during day, but for very short distances, with or without assistance. Spends majority of each shift in a bed or chair.

4. Walks frequently
Walks outside room at least twice a day and inside room at least once every two hours during waking hours.

3. Slightly limited
Makes frequent though slight changes in body or extremity position independently.

4. No limitations
Makes major and frequent changes in position without assistance.

3. Adequate
Eats over half of most meals. Eats a total of 4 servings of protein (meat, dairy products) per day. Occasionally will refuse a meal, but will usually take a supplement when offered.
OR
Is on a tube feeding or TPN regimen which probably meets most of nutritional needs.

4. Excellent
Eats most of every meal. Never refuses a meal. Usually eats a total of 4 or more servings of meat and dairy products. Occasionally eats between meals. Does not require supplementation.

The Braden scale is the most widely used scale in the United States for determining a patient's risk of pressure ulcers.

3. No apparent problem
Moves in bed and in chair independently and has sufficient muscle strength to lift up completely during move. Maintains good position in bed or chair.

Total score

Norton scale

Total the numbers from each category that describes your patient. A score of 14 or less indicates a risk of developing pressure ulcers.

Physical condition		Mental condition		Activity		Mobility		Incontinence		Total score
Good	4	Alert	4	Ambulatory	4	Full	4	None	4	
Fair	3	Apathetic	3	Walk/help	3	Slightly limited	3	Occasional	3	
Poor	2	Confused	2	Chairbound	2	Very limited	2	Usually-urine	2	Total
Very bad	1	Stuporous	1	Bedridden	1	Immobile	1	Urine/feces	1	score

Name: _____ Date: _____

Name: _____ Date: _____

Name: _____ Date: _____

> The Norton scale is another scale recommended to determine a patient's risk of pressure ulcers.

When to assess and reassess

How frequently you assess and reassess your patient for pressure ulcer risk will depend on the care setting. The Agency for Healthcare Research and Quality and the Wound, Ostomy, and Continence Nurses Society recommend the following intervals:

■ *Acute care:* Upon admission and then every 24 to 48 hours or when the patient's condition changes

■ *Long-term care:* Upon admission and then weekly for the first 4 weeks and monthly to quarterly after that; also whenever the patient's condition changes

■ *Home health care:* Upon admission and at every visit.

take note

Pressure ulcer documentation

01/16/07	1415	Nursing admit note: Received pt. from ED at 1300. Sacral pressure ulcer noted: 5½ cm length, 3 cm width, 0.4 cm depth. Tunneling present between 9 and 10 o'clock, measuring 2 cm in depth. Small amount of serosanguineous drainage oozing from wound bed. No odor present. Ulcer bed is red with granulation tissue. Thin band (approximately 0.5 cm) of yellow slough present around entire ulcer margin. Surrounding skin pink and intact, except for 1-cm area of induration at 4 o'clock. Pt. reported ulcer pain as 7 on 0-to-10 scale. Hydrocodone administered at 1330 per order. Pt. now reports pain as 3 on 0-to-10 scale. Wound/ostomy nurse N. Cooper paged to evaluate pt. and determine wound care plan. Wet-to-dry dressing applied and pt. positioned off of ulcer until evaluation. *L. Bradley, RN*

Prevention

> Preventing pressure ulcers—which includes identifying patients at risk and taking action to minimize those risks—is a major health care goal.

Managing the intensity and duration of pressure is key to preventing pressure ulcers, especially for patients with limited mobility. Other prevention strategies include reducing friction and shear, minimizing moisture, maximizing nutritional status, and controlling chronic illnesses that contribute to pressure ulcer development (such as diabetes).

Positioning patients

To position a reclining patient, use the Rule of 30 (raising the head of the bed 30 degrees, as shown below). Raising the head more than 30 degrees can cause shearing pressure. When you must raise it more (such as at mealtimes), keep the periods brief.

30°

When repositioning a patient from the left side to the right, make sure his weight rests on the buttock, not the hipbone. This reduces pressure on the trochanter and sacrum. The angle between the bed and an imaginary lateral line through the hips should be about 30 degrees (as shown here).

If needed, use pillows or a foam wedge to help the patient maintain the proper position. Cushion pressure points, such as the knees and shoulders, with pillows.

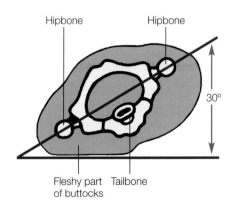

Hipbone   Hipbone

30°

Fleshy part   Tailbone
of buttocks

Pressure ulcer prevention algorithm

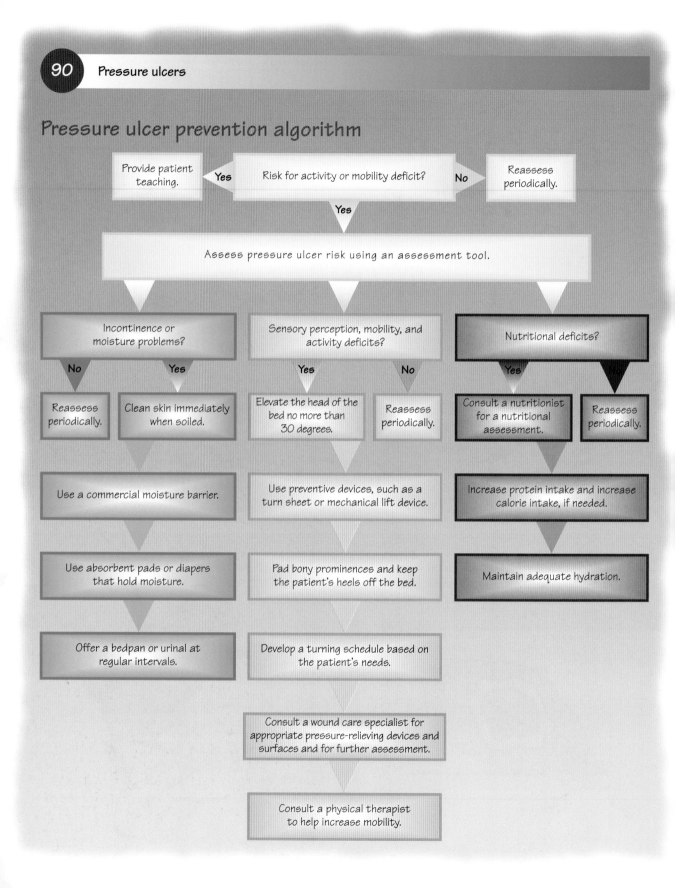

| Provide patient teaching. | ◄ Yes | Risk for activity or mobility deficit? | No ► | Reassess periodically. |

Yes ▼

Assess pressure ulcer risk using an assessment tool.

Incontinence or moisture problems?

No ◄   ► Yes

Reassess periodically.

Clean skin immediately when soiled.

Use a commercial moisture barrier.

Use absorbent pads or diapers that hold moisture.

Offer a bedpan or urinal at regular intervals.

Sensory perception, mobility, and activity deficits?

Yes ◄   ► No

Elevate the head of the bed no more than 30 degrees.

Reassess periodically.

Use preventive devices, such as a turn sheet or mechanical lift device.

Pad bony prominences and keep the patient's heels off the bed.

Develop a turning schedule based on the patient's needs.

Consult a wound care specialist for appropriate pressure-relieving devices and surfaces and for further assessment.

Consult a physical therapist to help increase mobility.

Nutritional deficits?

Yes

Consult a nutritionist for a nutritional assessment.

Reassess periodically.

Increase protein intake and increase calorie intake, if needed.

Maintain adequate hydration.

Comparing support surface characteristics

Characteristics	Support devices					
	Air-fluidized bed	*Low-air-loss bed*	*Alternating air mattress*	*Static flotation (air or water)*	*Foam overlay mattress*	*Standard mattress*
Increased support area	✔	✔	✔	✔	✔	✖
Low moisture retention	✔	✔	✖	✖	✖	✖
Reduced heat accumulation	✔	✔	✖	✖	✖	✖
Shear reduction	✔	??	✔	✔	✖	✖
Pressure redistribution	✔	✔	✔	✔	✔	✖
Dynamic	✔	✔	✔	✖	✖	✖
Cost per day	$$$$$	$$$$$	$$$	$	$	$

Air-fluidized therapy bed

The fluidlike surface of an air-fluidized therapy bed redistributes pressure on the skin, thereby helping prevent pressure ulcers and promote wound healing. The bed also provides the advantages of flotation without the disadvantages of instability, patient positioning difficulties, and immobility.

Key
Yes ✔
No ✖
Unknown ??
High cost $$$$$
Moderate cost $$$
Low cost $

> Just as actors need emotional support to combat psychological pressure, patients need physical support to combat pressure ulcers.

Monofilament polyester sheet allows for the passage of moisture

Air-fluidized chamber contains microspheres suspended in warm air that relieve pressure and eliminate shear and friction to trouble areas, such as the sacrum, ischium, and trochanter

Easy touch control panel

Low-air-loss therapy bed

Low-air-loss therapy beds contain segmented air cushions that inflate to help redistribute pressure on skin surfaces and to minimize shear forces during repositioning. The beds also circulate cool air to promote evaporation and temperature reduction, which helps prevent maceration. These mattresses fit on regular hospital bed frames.

Patient's body

Back

Buttocks

Legs

Mattress

Air- and vapor-permeable, water-resistant fabric covering helps reduce friction and shear

Air circulates through these cushions and conforms to the patient's body, evenly distributing pressure

Pressure control system

Air hose

Alternating pressure mattress

An alternating pressure mattress contains chambers filled with air or water that periodically circulates to create alternating low- and high-pressure areas. This action redistributes pressure while stimulating blood circulation.

Some alternating pressure mattress models also include low-air-loss therapy.

Air- and vapor-permeable, water-resistant fabric covering helps reduce friction and shear

Chambers filled with air or water alternately inflate and deflate to create high- and low-pressure areas

Electric pump circulates air or water

Using a hydraulic lift

Using a hydraulic lift to transfer an immobile or obese patient reduces the effects of shear and friction on the skin—a key strategy of pressure ulcer prevention. These general guidelines will help you to transfer your patient safely and comfortably. Be sure to follow the manufacturer's instructions.

After placing the patient in a supine position in the center of the sling, position the hydraulic lift above him (as shown below). Then attach the chains to the hooks on the sling.

Turn the lift handle clockwise to raise the patient to the sitting position. If he's positioned properly, continue to raise him until he's suspended just above the bed.

After positioning the patient above the wheelchair, turn the lift handle counterclockwise to lower him onto the seat. When the chains become slack, stop turning and unhook the sling from the lift.

> The Pressure Ulcer Scale for Healing (PUSH) tool can help you monitor, reassess, and document pressure ulcers.

Assessment

Assess pressure ulcers weekly. A well-vascularized pressure ulcer without infection should show signs of healing within 2 weeks. If not, reevaluate the care plan.

PUSH tool

Patient's name: _____ Patient ID #: _____

Ulcer location: _____ Date: _____

Directions

Observe and measure the pressure ulcer. Categorize the ulcer with respect to surface area, exudate, and type of wound tissue. Record a subscore for each of the ulcer characteristics. Add the subscores to obtain the total score. A comparison of total scores measured over time provides an indication of the improvement or deterioration in pressure ulcer healing.

Length × width

0 cm^2	1 < 0.3 cm^2	2 0.3 to 0.6 cm^2	3 0.7 to 1 cm^2	4 1.1 to 2 cm^2	5 2.1 to 3 cm^2	Subscore
	6 3.1 to 4 cm^2	7 4.1 to 8 cm^2	8 8.1 to 12 cm^2	9 12.1 to 24 cm^2	10 > 24 cm^2	

Exudate amount

0 None	1 Light	2 Moderate	3 Heavy	–	–	Subscore

Tissue type

0 Closed	1 Epithelial tissue	2 Granulation tissue	3 Slough	4 Necrotic tissue	–	Subscore

Total score

Length × width

Measure the greatest length (head-to-toe) and the greatest width (side-to-side) using a centimeter ruler. Multiply these two measurements (length × width) to obtain an estimate of surface area in square centimeters (cm^2). Don't guess! Always use a centimeter ruler and always use the same method each time you measure.

Exudate amount

Estimate the amount of exudate (drainage) present after removing the dressing and before applying any topical agent to the ulcer. Estimate as none, light, moderate, or heavy.

Tissue type

This refers to the types of tissue in the wound bed. Score as a 4 if you note necrotic tissue. Score as a 3 if you observe slough but no necrotic tissue. Score a clean wound that contains granulation tissue as a 2. Score a superficial wound that's reepithelializing as a 1. When the wound is closed, score it as a 0. The following guide describes each tissue type:

4—Necrotic tissue (eschar): Black, brown, or tan tissue that adheres firmly to the wound bed or ulcer edges and may be either firmer or softer than surrounding tissue

3—Slough: Yellow or white tissue that adheres to the ulcer bed in strings or thick clumps or is mucinous

2—Granulation tissue: Pink or beefy red tissue with a shiny, moist, granular appearance

1—Epithelial tissue: For superficial ulcers, new pink or shiny tissue (skin) that grows in from the edges or as islands on the ulcer surface

0—Closed or resurfaced: Completely covered wound with epithelium (new skin).

Staging

Pressure ulcer staging reflects the depth and extent of tissue involvement. The classification system developed by the National Pressure Ulcer Advisory Panel (NPUAP) is the most widely used system for staging pressure ulcers. The NPUAP recently redefined its pressure ulcer stages by adding two new stages for deep tissue injury and unstageable ulcers.

Stage I

Stage I ulcers are characterized by intact skin with nonblanchable redness of a localized area, usually over a bony prominence. Darkly pigmented skin may not have visible blanching, but its color may differ from the surrounding area.

To identify a stage I pressure ulcer, compare the suspected area to an adjacent area or to the same region on the other side of the body. Indications of a stage I pressure ulcer include differences in:

- skin temperature (warmth or coolness)
- tissue consistency (firm)
- sensation (pain).

Suspected deep tissue injury

Deep tissue injury is characterized by a purple or maroon localized area of intact skin or blood-filled blister caused by damage of underlying soft tissue from pressure or shear. The injury may be preceded by tissue that's painful, firm, mushy, boggy, or warm or cool compared to adjacent tissue. It may be difficult to detect in individuals with dark skin tones.

Reddened area —
— Epidermis
— Dermis
— Subcutaneous tissue
— Muscle
— Bone

Stage II

A stage II pressure ulcer is characterized by partial-thickness loss of the dermis, presenting as a shallow, open ulcer with a red-pink wound bed without slough. It may also present as an intact or open serum-filled blister.

Stage III

A stage III pressure ulcer is characterized by full-thickness tissue loss. Subcutaneous fat may be visible, but bone, tendon, and muscle aren't exposed. Slough may be present but doesn't obscure the depth of tissue loss. Undermining and tunneling may be present. The depth of a stage III ulcer varies by anatomical location.

— Epidermis

— Dermis

— Subcutaneous tissue

— Muscle

— Bone

All the world's a stage... at least as far as pressure ulcers go.

Stage IV

A stage IV pressure ulcer involves full-thickness tissue loss with exposed bone, tendon, or muscle. Slough or eschar may be present on some parts of the wound bed. Undermining and tunneling are also common. The depth of a stage IV ulcer varies by anatomical location.

- Epidermis
- Dermis
- Subcutaneous tissue
- Muscle
- Bone

Alas, some pressure ulcers are unstageable until slough and eschar are removed.

Unstageable

An unstageable ulcer is characterized by full-thickness tissue loss in which the base of the ulcer in the wound bed is covered by slough (yellow, tan, gray, green, or brown), eschar (tan, brown, or black), or both. Until enough slough or eschar is removed to expose the base of the wound, the true depth, and therefore stage, can't be determined.

Treatment

Treatment of pressure ulcers includes nutritional assessment and support, management of tissue loads, ulcer care, and management of bacterial colonization and infection.

Management of pressure ulcers algorithm

1 Pressure ulcer identification

2 Initial assessment

3 Education and development of treatment plan

4 Nutritional assessment and support (see page 100)

5 Management of tissue loads (see page 101)

6 Ulcer care; managing bacterial colonization and infection (see page 102)

7 Is ulcer healing?

Yes

No

8 Monitor

9 Reassessment of treatment plan and evaluation of adherence

Return to 3

 Key

Yes-no decision
Interventions
Education and counseling
Refer to previous node

Nutritional assessment and support algorithm

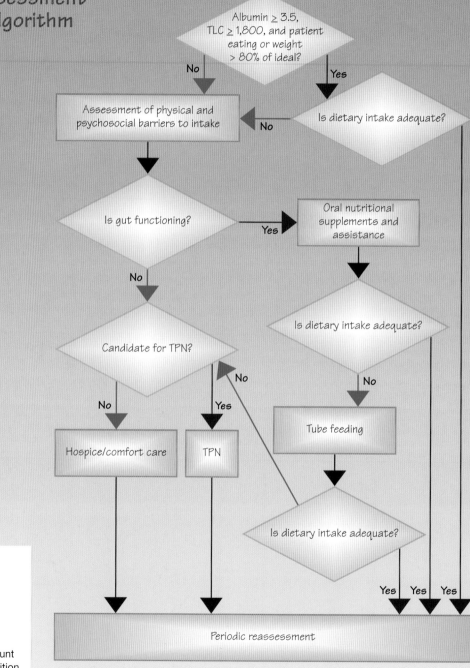

Key

◇ Yes-no decision
▭ Interventions

Note:
TLC = Total lymphocyte count
TPN = Total parenteral nutrition

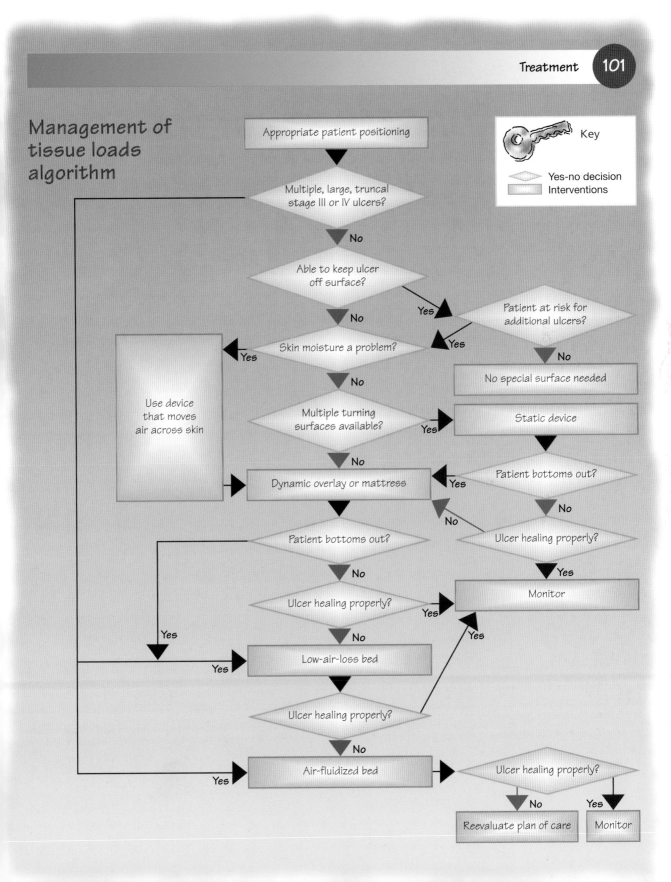

Management of tissue loads algorithm

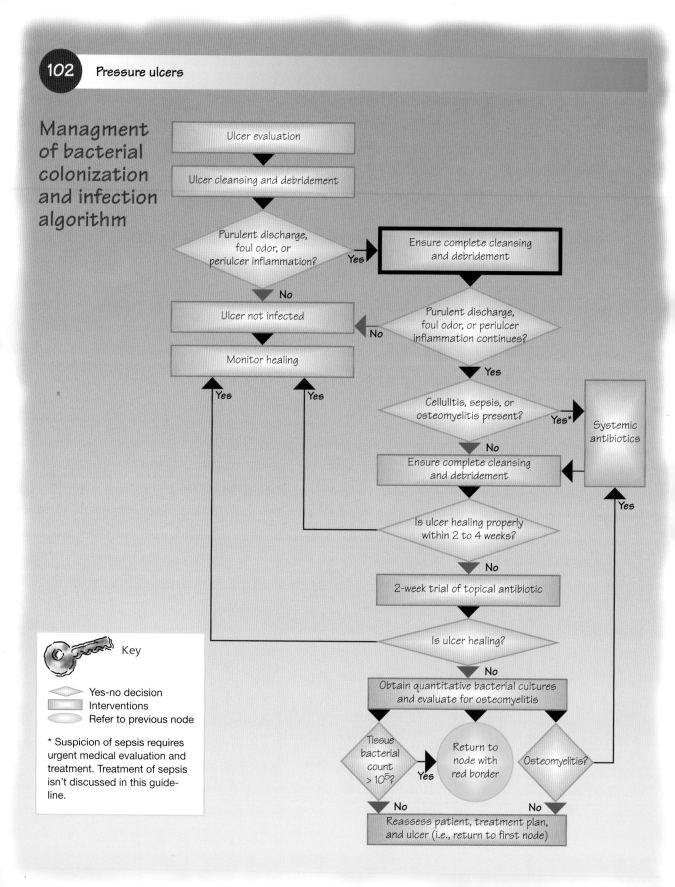

Managment of bacterial colonization and infection algorithm

Ulcer evaluation

Ulcer cleansing and debridement

Purulent discharge, foul odor, or periulcer inflammation?

Yes → Ensure complete cleansing and debridement

No

Ulcer not infected

Monitor healing

Purulent discharge, foul odor, or periulcer inflammation continues?

No

Yes

Cellulitis, sepsis, or osteomyelitis present?

Yes* → Systemic antibiotics

No

Ensure complete cleansing and debridement

Is ulcer healing properly within 2 to 4 weeks?

Yes

No

2-week trial of topical antibiotic

Is ulcer healing?

Yes

No

Obtain quantitative bacterial cultures and evaluate for osteomyelitis

Tissue bacterial count > 10^5?

Yes → Return to node with red border

Osteomyelitis?

Yes

No

No

Reassess patient, treatment plan, and ulcer (i.e., return to first node)

Key

Yes-no decision
Interventions
Refer to previous node

* Suspicion of sepsis requires urgent medical evaluation and treatment. Treatment of sepsis isn't discussed in this guide-line.

Pressure ulcer care

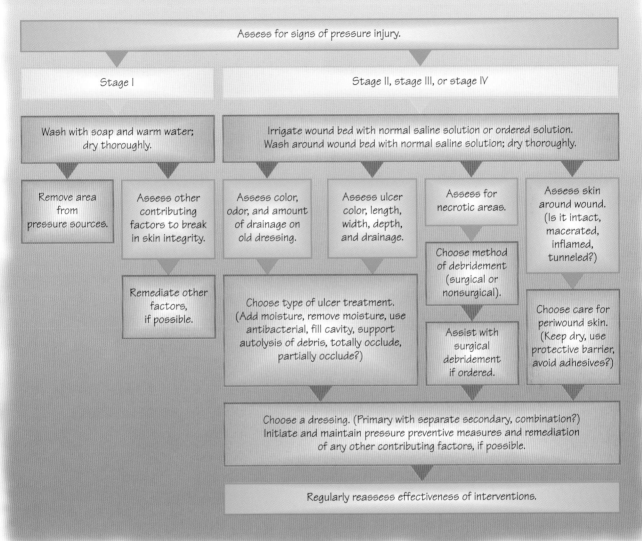

Assess for signs of pressure injury.

Stage I

Stage II, stage III, or stage IV

Wash with soap and warm water; dry thoroughly.

Irrigate wound bed with normal saline solution or ordered solution.
Wash around wound bed with normal saline solution; dry thoroughly.

Remove area from pressure sources.

Assess other contributing factors to break in skin integrity.

Assess color, odor, and amount of drainage on old dressing.

Assess ulcer color, length, width, depth, and drainage.

Assess for necrotic areas.

Assess skin around wound. (Is it intact, macerated, inflamed, tunneled?)

Remediate other factors, if possible.

Choose type of ulcer treatment. (Add moisture, remove moisture, use antibacterial, fill cavity, support autolysis of debris, totally occlude, partially occlude?)

Choose method of debridement (surgical or nonsurgical).

Assist with surgical debridement if ordered.

Choose care for periwound skin. (Keep dry, use protective barrier, avoid adhesives?)

Choose a dressing. (Primary with separate secondary, combination?)
Initiate and maintain pressure preventive measures and remediation of any other contributing factors, if possible.

Regularly reassess effectiveness of interventions.

Matchmaker

Match the four illustrations of pressure ulcers with their correct stage.

1. ___

2. ___

A. Stage I
B. Stage II
C. Stage III
D. Stage IV

3. ___

4. ___

Able to label?

Label the pressure points susceptible to ulcer formation in the illustration.

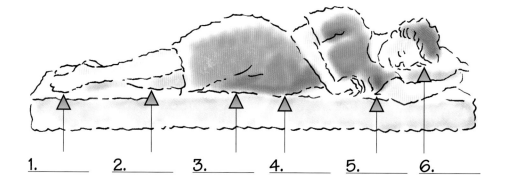

1. _____ 2. _____ 3. _____ 4. _____ 5. _____ 6. _____

Answers: Matchmaker 1. B, 2. A, 3. D, 4. C; Able to label? 1. Sides of feet and ankles, 2. Front of knee, 3. Upper thighbone, 4. Upper hipbone, 5. Shoulder, 6. Side of head.

7
Vascular ulcers

An ulcer by any other name...just might be a vascular ulcer.

Vascular system

The body's vascular system consists of:
- veins (carry blood toward the heart)
- arteries (carry blood away from the heart)
- lymphatic system (a separate circulatory system that collects waste products and delivers them to the venous system).

Veins

Veins carry deoxygenated blood back to the heart for reoxygenation.

A close look at a vein

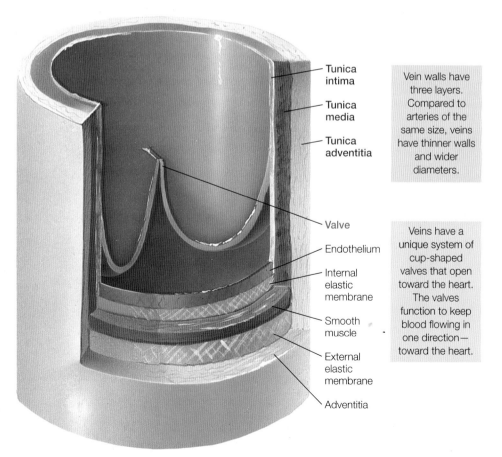

Tunica intima

Tunica media

Tunica adventitia

Valve

Endothelium

Internal elastic membrane

Smooth muscle

External elastic membrane

Adventitia

Vein walls have three layers. Compared to arteries of the same size, veins have thinner walls and wider diameters.

Veins have a unique system of cup-shaped valves that open toward the heart. The valves function to keep blood flowing in one direction—toward the heart.

Major lower limb veins

Venous ulcers most commonly occur in the lower extremities. The illustration below shows the major veins in this part of the body.

Types of veins

The lower portion of the body contains three major types of veins.

Superficial veins

Superficial veins lie just beneath the skin; they drain through perforator veins into deep veins.

Perforator veins

Perforator veins connect superficial to deep veins.

Deep veins

Deep veins receive venous blood from perforator veins and return it to the heart.

He's really a superficial vein. He just thinks if he reads enough literature, people will start to think he's deep.

The Heart Is A Lonely Hunter

Abdominal vena cava

Common iliac vein

Inferior epigastric vein

Superficial circumflex iliac vein

Superficial epigastric vein

Internal iliac vein

External iliac vein

Great saphenous vein

Popliteal vein

Femoral vein

Deep veins of the knee

Superficial veins of the thigh and knee

Popliteal vein

Small saphenous vein

Fibular vein

Posterior tibial vein

Great saphenous vein

Deep veins of the foot

Superficial veins of the anterior foot

Arteries

Arteries carry blood from the heart to every functioning cell in the body. The lower portion of the body receives its arterial flow through the abdominal aorta and the major arteries branching from it.

A close look at an artery

Tunica
intima

Tunica
media

Tunica
adventitia

Endothelium

Internal
elastic
membrane

Smooth
muscle

External
elastic
membrane

Adventitia

Like vein walls, artery walls have three layers.

An artery's strong, muscular walls allow it to expand and relax with each heartbeat.

Major lower limb arteries

Arterial ulcers most commonly occur in the lower extremities. This illustration identifies the major arteries in the lower portion of the body.

Superficial circumflex iliac artery

Medial femoral circumflex artery

Lateral femoral circumflex artery

Perforating branch

Medial superior genicular artery

Medial inferior genicular artery

Lateral plantar artery

Deep plantar arterial arch

Dorsal metatarsal arteries

Dorsal digital arteries

Aorta

Gonadal artery

Common iliac artery

Internal iliac artery

External iliac artery

Femoral artery

Deep femoral artery

Descending genicular artery

Lateral superior genicular artery

Popliteal artery

Lateral inferior genicular artery

Anterior tibial artery

Peroneal artery

Posterior tibial artery

Dorsalis pedis artery

Lateral tarsal artery

Arcuate artery

Assessing lower extremity pulses

Assessing pulses is an effective way to evaluate arterial blood flow to the lower extremities. These illustrations show where to position your fingers when palpating for pulses of the lower extremities. Use your index and middle fingers to apply pressure.

Femoral pulse

Press relatively hard at a point inferior to the inguinal ligament. For obese patients, palpate in the groin crease, halfway between the pubic bone and hip bone.

Popliteal pulse

Press firmly in the popliteal fossa at the back of the knee.

Dorsalis pedis pulse

Place your fingers on the medial dorsum of the foot while the patient points his toes down. The pulse is difficult to palpate here and may seem absent in healthy patients.

Posterior tibial pulse

Apply pressure behind and slightly below the medial malleolus.

Lymphatic system

The lymphatic system is a vascular network that drains lymph (a protein-rich fluid similar to plasma) from body tissues and intravascular compartments and returns it to the venous system.

Lymphatic system and drainage route

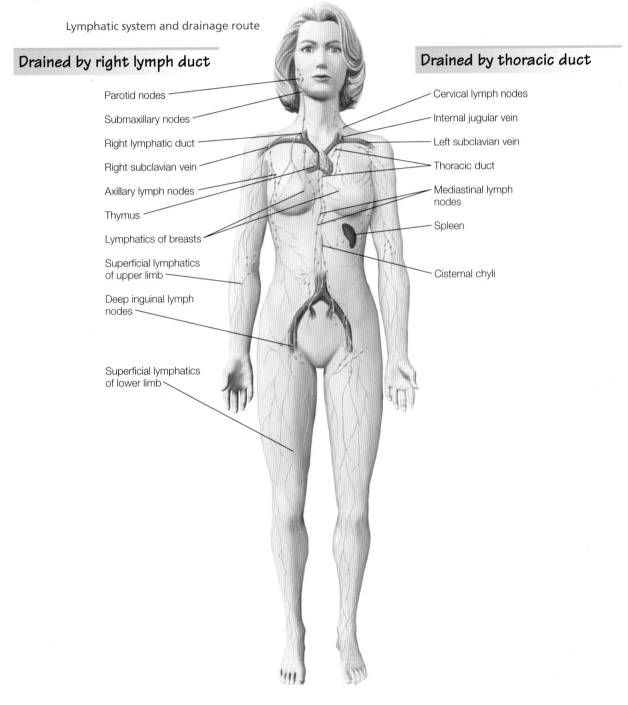

Drained by right lymph duct

Parotid nodes

Submaxillary nodes

Right lymphatic duct

Right subclavian vein

Axillary lymph nodes

Thymus

Lymphatics of breasts

Superficial lymphatics of upper limb

Deep inguinal lymph nodes

Superficial lymphatics of lower limb

Drained by thoracic duct

Cervical lymph nodes

Internal jugular vein

Left subclavian vein

Thoracic duct

Mediastinal lymph nodes

Spleen

Cisternal chyli

The lymphatic system begins peripherally, with lymph capillaries that absorb fluid. The capillaries proceed centrally to thin vascular vessels. These vessels empty into collecting ducts, which empty into major veins at the base of the neck.

Vascular ulcers

Disorders of the venous, arterial, and lymphatic systems can cause chronic wounds, called *vascular ulcers*, to develop.

> Venous and arterial ulcers tend to occur on the distal portion of the legs, whereas lymphatic ulcers occur on either the arms or the legs.

Types of vascular ulcers

Type of ulcer	Typical location	Clinical findings
Venous	▪ Anywhere from ankle to midcalf ▪ Most common on medial aspect of ankle above the malleolus	▪ Irregular shape ▪ Dry, crusted or moist, slightly macerated borders ▪ Shallow wound base covered with beefy red granulation tissue, yellow film, or gray necrotic tissue (black necrotic tissue rarely present except in acute injury) ▪ Edema (one of the first signs of venous disease) ▪ Hyperpigmentation in calves due to buildup of hemosiderin (results from breakdown of red blood cells that have leaked into tissue) ▪ Atrophie blanche (spots of ivory white plaque in skin, usually surrounded by hyperpigmentation)
Arterial	▪ Tips of toes, corners of nail beds on toes, over bony prominences, and between toes	▪ Well-demarcated wound edges ▪ Pale and dry wound base with no granulation tissue (due to impaired blood flow to tissue) ▪ Surrounding skin that feels cooler than normal on palpation ▪ Dependent rubor (ischemic skin becomes deep red when patient places his foot in a dependent position) ▪ Thin, pale yellow nails (may be thickened as a result of fungal infection) ▪ History of claudication (pain distal to a narrowed artery brought on by exercise and relieved by rest) and rest pain (commonly occurs in foot when patient is asleep; alleviated by lowering extremity)
Lymphatic	▪ Arms and legs, most commonly ankle area	▪ Shallow ulcer bed that may be oozing, moist, or blistered ▪ Firm, fibrotic surrounding skin that's thickened by edema ▪ Cellulitis (possibly)

Between 70% and 90% of all leg ulcers are venous ulcers.

Venous ulcers

When leg veins fail to propel a sufficient supply of blood back to the heart, blood begins to pool in the legs (venous insufficiency). Causes of venous insufficiency include:

■ **incompetent valves**—most common cause; can result when a blood clot disrupts valve function or when a vein distends to the point that the valve no longer closes completely

■ **inadequate calf muscle function.**

Signs of venous insufficiency

Physical activity is crucial to adequate venous return. Leg muscle paralysis or prolonged inactivity can drastically hinder the amount of blood returning to the heart.

Pitting edema (making it difficult to find pulse)

Brown pigment (hemosiderin stain)

Ulcer around ankle

Other signs and symptoms of venous insufficiency

■ Fibrotic skin
A buildup of fibrin causes skin and subcutaneous tissue to thicken and become fibrotic—a condition called *lipodermatosclerosis*. The skin eventually develops a shiny, taut appearance.

■ Eczema
Eczema (venous dermatitis) commonly occurs, particularly in patients with recurrent ulcers. Skin over scar tissue and edematous tissue is fragile. Drainage from larger ulcers—or medications themselves—can irritate the skin and aggravate eczema.

A closer look at venous ulcers

Venous ulcers most commonly occur above the medial malleolus. These ulcers have irregular borders and typically appear moist.

Distended
leg veins

Venous dermatitis

Irregular
border

Hemosiderosis

Hemosiderosis

Lipodermatosclerosis

Venous dermatitis

Note the common characteristics of venous ulcers in these photographs: moist, beefy red wound base; hemosiderosis; and lipodermatosclerosis.

Moist, beefy red wound base

Lipodermatosclerosis

Hemosiderosis

Arterial ulcers

Also called *ischemic ulcers*, arterial ulcers result from tissue ischemia caused by insufficient blood flow through an artery (arterial insufficiency). Causes of arterial insufficiency include arterial stenosis (narrowing) or obstruction (from thrombosis, emboli, atherosclerosis, vasculitis, or Raynaud's phenomenon). Arterial ulcers most commonly occur in the area around the toes.

Development of an arterial ulcer

1 Arterial flow is diminished.

2 Trauma occurs to an area with arterial insufficiency.

3 Reduced blood flow impairs healing, and a chronic wound results.

The most common cause of arterial ulcers is atherosclerosis, so stay back plaque.

Understanding atherosclerosis

In atherosclerosis, fatty, fibrous plaques progressively narrow the arterial lumen. This reduces blood flow and leads to tissue ischemia. The illustrations below show the progression of atherosclerosis.

Normal artery

Fatty streak

Reduced blood flow

Fibrous plaque

Severely restricted blood flow

Fibrous plaque

Risk factors for atherosclerosis

- Advanced age
- Smoking
- Obesity
- Hyperlipidemia
- Diabetes mellitus
- Hypertension
- Sedentary lifestyle

Signs of arterial insufficiency

Pale, shiny skin

Pain in legs and feet

Ulcer

Thick, ridged nails

Faint or absent pulses

Identifying dependent rubor

Dependent rubor is a sign of chronic arterial insufficiency. To elicit this sign during a physical examination:

■ Elevate the foot with the ulcer to a 30-degree angle. If the foot is ischemic, the skin will pale.

■ Ask the patient to lower the foot into a dependent position. Ischemic skin becomes deep red as the tissue fills with blood. This dramatic color change—called *dependent rubor*—signifies severe tissue ischemia.

Rubor

A closer look at arterial ulcers

Arterial ulcers have well-demarcated edges. Because of decreased blood flow, the base of the ulcer is typically pale and dry and granulation tissue may be absent. On examination, you may notice an area of wet necrosis or a dry scab. The skin surrounding the ulcer will feel cooler than normal.

Common sites of arterial ulcers include the tips of the toes, the corners of nail beds on the toes, over bony prominences, and between toes.

Arterial toe ulcer

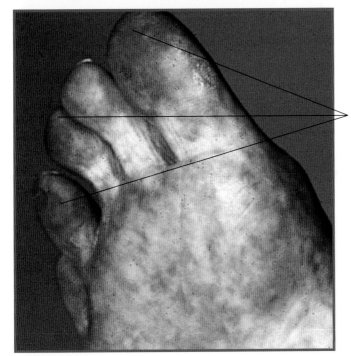

Ulcers resulting from arterial emboli

Lymphatic ulcers

Lymphatic ulcers result when a part of the body afflicted with lymphedema suffers an injury. Here are some predisposing factors for ulcer formation:

■ **Pressure on capillaries**—The skin and underlying tissue in areas with lymphedema become firm and fibrotic over time. This thickened tissue presses on capillaries, occluding blood flow and leaving the area vulnerable to ulcer formation. Because of the poor circulation, these ulcers are extremely difficult to treat.

■ **Skin folds from massive swelling**—Skin folds can trap moisture, leading to tissue maceration and ulcer formation.

■ **Traumatic injury or pressure**—Pressure or injury in an area with lymphedema commonly leads to an ulcer.

> Lymphatic ulcers commonly occur in the ankle area, but they can develop at any site of traumatic injury in an area with lymphedema.

Understanding lymphedema

Lymphedema occurs when an obstruction in the lymphatic system causes lymphatic fluid to build up in the interstitial spaces of body tissues. In the legs, the steady seepage of fluid into interstitial tissues can result in massive edema, as shown here.

Edema

Signs of lymphedema

- No pitting
- Thickened skin
- Swelling

A closer look at lymphatic ulcers

Lymphatic ulcers are typically shallow and may be oozing, moist, or blistered. The surrounding skin is usually firm, fibrotic, and thickened by edema. Cellulitis (tissue inflammation) may also be present.

Shallow, moist lymphatic ulcer

Treatment

Effective treatment of a vascular ulcer involves caring for the wound as well as managing the underlying vascular disease. The goals and treatment recommendations vary depending on the type of ulcer.

Type of ulcer	Treatment goals	Therapies and procedures	Wound care
Venous	■ Control edema ■ Manage underlying venous disease ■ Provide appropriate wound care	■ Limb elevation to allow gravity to drain fluid from the limb ■ Compression bandages, layered compression bandages, elastic bandages, compression pumps, compression stockings, or graduated compression support hosiery to reduce edema ■ Unna's boot to provide compression, protection, and a moist environment for healing	■ Apply occlusive dressings to promote moist wound healing, growth of granulation tissue, and reepithelialization. ■ Apply growth factors to the wound bed, as ordered, to improve healing rate. ■ Consider application of Apligraf (a bioengineered skin equivalent) for a venous ulcer that fails to heal within 4 weeks of treatment.
Arterial	■ Reestablish arterial flow ■ Provide appropriate wound care	■ Arterial bypass to restore arterial flow ■ Angioplasty (with possible stent insertion) to treat arterial stenosis	■ Keep the wound dry and protected from pressure. ■ As ordered, apply an antiseptic or antimicrobial agent and then place small gauze pads between the toes. Change the pads daily to keep toe ulcers dry. ■ Never soak arterial ulcers. ■ If revascularization succeeds, change the type of dressing to keep moist tissue moist and dry tissue dry.
Lymphatic	■ Reduce edema ■ Prevent infection ■ Provide appropriate wound care	■ Limb elevation and compression pump therapy to reduce edema ■ Comprehensive decongestive therapy (a form of massage) to reduce edema and improve circulation	■ Follow guidelines for venous ulcer care. ■ Choose dressings that can manage large fluid loads while protecting the surrounding skin, such as foams and other absorbent dressings.

Treatment of venous ulcers algorithm

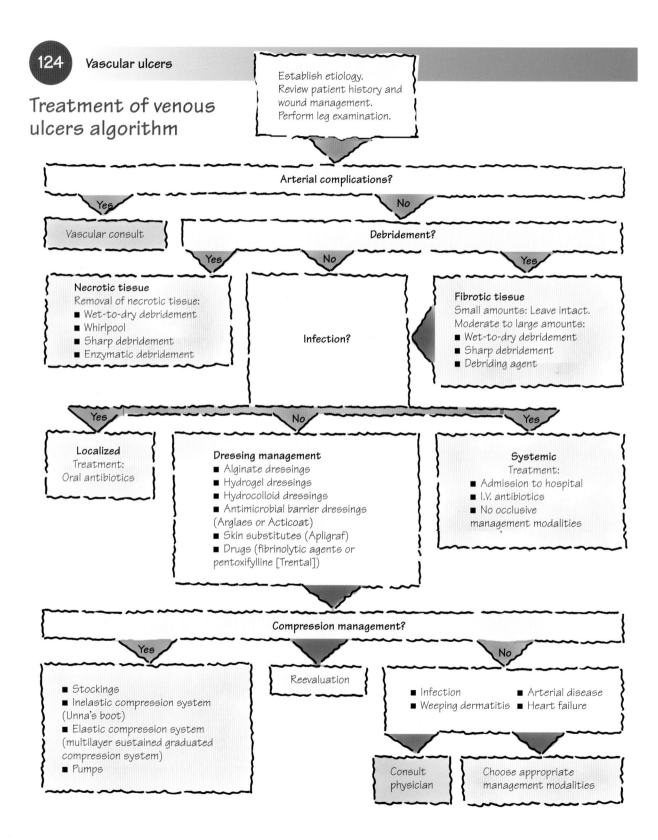

Establish etiology.
Review patient history and wound management.
Perform leg examination.

Arterial complications?

Yes → Vascular consult

No → **Debridement?**

Yes →
Necrotic tissue
Removal of necrotic tissue:
- Wet-to-dry debridement
- Whirlpool
- Sharp debridement
- Enzymatic debridement

No → **Infection?**

Yes →
Fibrotic tissue
Small amounts: Leave intact.
Moderate to large amounts:
- Wet-to-dry debridement
- Sharp debridement
- Debriding agent

Yes →
Localized
Treatment:
Oral antibiotics

No →
Dressing management
- Alginate dressings
- Hydrogel dressings
- Hydrocolloid dressings
- Antimicrobial barrier dressings (Arglaes or Acticoat)
- Skin substitutes (Apligraf)
- Drugs (fibrinolytic agents or pentoxifylline [Trental])

Yes →
Systemic
Treatment:
- Admission to hospital
- I.V. antibiotics
- No occlusive management modalities

Compression management?

Yes →
- Stockings
- Inelastic compression system (Unna's boot)
- Elastic compression system (multilayer sustained graduated compression system)
- Pumps

Reevaluation

No →
- Infection
- Weeping dermatitis
- Arterial disease
- Heart failure

Consult physician

Choose appropriate management modalities

> A treatment for venous ulcers involves applying an inelastic compression system called Unna's boot.

How to wrap Unna's boot

■ Clean the patient's skin thoroughly.

■ Flex the patient's knee.

■ With the foot positioned at a right angle to the leg, wrap the medicated gauze bandage firmly—not tightly—around the patient's foot. Make sure the dressing covers the heel.

■ Continue wrapping upward, overlapping the layers by 50% with each turn. Make sure the dressing circles the leg at an angle to avoid compromising the circulation. Smooth the boot with your free hand as you go, as shown below.

■ Stop wrapping about 1″ (2.5 cm) below the knee, as shown below. If constriction develops as the dressing hardens, make a 2″ (5.1-cm) slit in the boot just below the knee.

■ If drainage is excessive, wrap a roller gauze dressing over the boot.

■ Finally, wrap the boot with an elastic bandage in a figure-eight pattern, as shown below.

take note

Documenting Unna's boot application

| 1/2/07 | 1030 | Unna's boot applied to pt's right leg at 0930. Ulcer above right medial malleolus measures 3 cm length, 1.5 cm width, 0.2 cm depth. Wound bed appears moist and beefy red. No drainage or odor noted. Surrounding skin dry and scaly but intact. Right lower extremity pulses easily palpable. Wound cleaned with NSS and allowed to dry thoroughly. Medicated gauze bandage applied on right leg from just above the toes to the knee, then covered with elastic bandage. Assisted patient in elevation of right leg to allow for drying. Toes on right foot presently appear pink with immediate capillary refill, no edema, normal sensation. Pt. tolerated procedure well. ———— Isa Rapp, R.N. |

Treatment of arterial ulcers algorithm

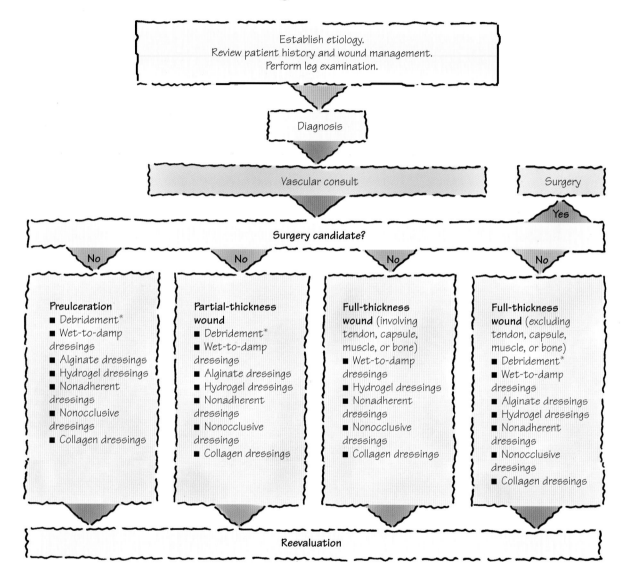

Establish etiology.
Review patient history and wound management.
Perform leg examination.

Diagnosis

Vascular consult

Surgery

Yes

Surgery candidate?

No   No   No   No

Preulceration
■ Debridement*
■ Wet-to-damp dressings
■ Alginate dressings
■ Hydrogel dressings
■ Nonadherent dressings
■ Nonocclusive dressings
■ Collagen dressings

Partial-thickness wound
■ Debridement*
■ Wet-to-damp dressings
■ Alginate dressings
■ Hydrogel dressings
■ Nonadherent dressings
■ Nonocclusive dressings
■ Collagen dressings

Full-thickness wound (involving tendon, capsule, muscle, or bone)
■ Wet-to-damp dressings
■ Hydrogel dressings
■ Nonadherent dressings
■ Nonocclusive dressings
■ Collagen dressings

Full-thickness wound (excluding tendon, capsule, muscle, or bone)
■ Debridement*
■ Wet-to-damp dressings
■ Alginate dressings
■ Hydrogel dressings
■ Nonadherent dressings
■ Nonocclusive dressings
■ Collagen dressings

Reevaluation

* Debride only arterial ulcers with necrotic tissue. Be careful not to disturb the already compromised arteries.

Best dressed

Dressings for vascular ulcers

Dressing	Indications and contraindications		
	VENOUS ULCERS	ARTERIAL ULCERS	LYMPHATIC ULCERS
Alginate	• Use to manage copious drainage.	• Use isn't indicated.	• Use for heavily draining wounds.
Foam	• Use to protect the ulcer. • Use for absorption underneath a compression dressing.	• Use to protect the ulcer. • Use with dry gangrene. • Use for a moist, revascularized ulcer.	• Use to protect the ulcer. • Use to absorb drainage.
Gauze	• Use for absorption.	• Use for protection and to allow dry gangrene to maintain its dryness.	• Use for absorption or padding (don't allow it to dry out on the ulcer).
Hydrocolloid	• Use to promote granulation. • Use to manage pain. • Don't use when copious drainage is present.	• Use for autolytic debridement. • Use for primary dressing after revascularization. • Don't use on ischemic tissue. • Don't use when infection or cellulitis is present.	• Use to protect the skin. • Use to promote epithelialization. • Don't use when copious drainage is present. • Don't use when cellulitis is present.
Hydrogel	• Don't use when copious drainage is present.	• Use to maintain a moist wound bed. • Use to debride.	• Use to manage pain. • Use to debride.
Transparent film	• Use isn't indicated.	• Use only after the ulcer has almost completely healed.	• Use to protect fragile skin.

Matchmaker

Match the three types of ulcers shown here with their names.

1. _____ 2. _____ 3. _____

A. Arterial ulcer
B. Lymphatic ulcer
C. Venous ulcer

My word!

Use the clues to help you unscramble the names of the major cause of each type of vascular ulcer. Then use the circled letters to answer the question posed.

Question: **What is the most common type of vascular ulcer?**

1. **What disorder is the major cause of arterial ulcers?**

cherriesalossto

— — — — — — — — — — —Ⓞ— —Ⓞ

2. **What disorder is the major cause of venous ulcers?**

conceiveiffunnyisus

Ⓞ— — —Ⓞ—   —Ⓞ— — — — — — — — — —

3. **What disorder is the major cause of lymphatic ulcers?**

playmedhem

— — — — —Ⓞ— — — —

8
Diabetic foot ulcers

Here's another take on ulcers...this time it's diabetic foot ulcers.

Causes

About 20.8 million people in the United States have diabetes. Of those, 15% will develop diabetic foot ulcers.

Diabetes mellitus—a metabolic disorder characterized by hyperglycemia—occurs because of a lack of insulin, a lack of insulin effect, or both. The high plasma glucose levels resulting from diabetes commonly damage blood vessels and nerves, leading to poor circulation and decreased sensation. This typically occurs in the lower extremities, leaving patients with diabetes at risk for developing foot ulcers.

Understanding diabetic trineuropathy

Uncontrolled diabetes commonly results in three concurrent neuropathies that dramatically increase a patient's risk of developing diabetic foot ulcers.

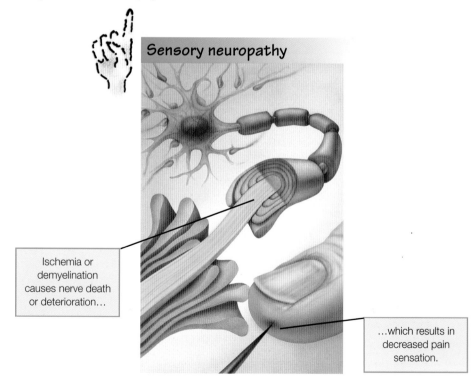

Sensory neuropathy

Ischemia or demyelination causes nerve death or deterioration…

…which results in decreased pain sensation.

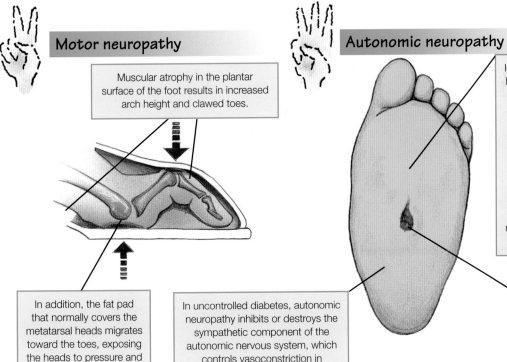

KEY PLAYERS IN DIABETIC FOOT ULCERS

■ **Diabetic neuropathy:** a nerve disorder causing impaired or lost function in tissue served by affected nerve fibers
■ **Pressure, friction, and shear:** pressure and mechanical forces that can lead to foot ulcers in patients with neuropathy
■ **Peripheral vascular disease:** disorder that impairs healing of existing ulcers and can also contribute to neuropathy

Motor neuropathy

Muscular atrophy in the plantar surface of the foot results in increased arch height and clawed toes.

In addition, the fat pad that normally covers the metatarsal heads migrates toward the toes, exposing the heads to pressure and increasing ulcer risk.

Autonomic neuropathy

In Charcot's disease, bones weakened by osteopenia suffer fractures that the patient doesn't feel because of sensory neuropathy. Over time, this process causes bony dissolution that culminates with the collapse of the midfoot into a rocker bottom deformity.

In uncontrolled diabetes, autonomic neuropathy inhibits or destroys the sympathetic component of the autonomic nervous system, which controls vasoconstriction in peripheral blood vessels. The resulting unfettered flow of blood to the lower limbs and feet may cause osteopenia in foot and ankle bones.

Midfoot ulcers that result from increased plantar pressure over the rocker bottom deformity heal more slowly than ulcers on the forefoot.

Performing the Semmes-Weinstein test

In the Semmes-Weinstein test, the practitioner uses a special monofilament to assess protective sensation in the feet of a patient with diabetes. This test helps to identify the degree of sensory neuropathy.

Performing the test

■ Ask the patient to close his eyes.
■ Ask the patient to identify where and when he feels the monofilament touch.
■ Place the 10-g monofilament on one of the testing points shown at right, and exert enough pressure to bow the monofilament.

Plantar surface of the first, third, and fifth toes

First, third, and fifth metatarsal heads

Bowed monofilament

Lateral and medial midfoot

Midheel

Middorsal surface of the foot

Take a bow. When performing the Semmes-Weinstein test, the monofilament should bow as shown in this illustration.

Characteristics

Diabetic foot ulcers commonly develop under a bony prominence, such as the one shown here under the metatarsal head of the great toe.

Impaired circulation and sensory neuropathy set the stage for ulcers to develop. These conditions allow excessive, repetitive pressure on the soles of the feet to go unchecked, commonly leading to an ulcer.

Epidermis

Dermis

Subcutaneous tissue

Muscle

Bone

Characteristics of skin surrounding a diabetic foot ulcer

Calluses
(considered
prewounds)

Erythema (indicates
inflammation or
infection)

Induration
(hardened edges)

Blood blisters
(hemorrhage
beneath a callus)

Skin fissures
(portals for
bacterial entry)

Dry, scaly skin

take note

Documenting a diabetic foot ulcer

2/28/07	1430	Dressing changed on diabetic foot ulcer on Ⓛ heel.
		Ulcer measures 2 cm length, 3 cm width, 0.5 cm
		depth. No drainage or odor noted. Site cleaned
		with NSS and allowed to dry thoroughly. Wound
		bed appears moist and pink with a thin ring of
		yellow slough at edges. Calloused border noted at
		wound edge from 6 o'clock to 8 o'clock. Hydrogel
		applied to site and dressed per physician order.
		Maintaining heels off bed, using blankets to
		elevate. Patient tolerated procedure well; states
		pain as 1 on a 0-to-10 scale before and after
		procedure. ———— *Diane Bettick, R.N.*

Ulcer location	Characteristics
Plantar surface	Even wound margins
Great toe	Deep wound bed
Metatarsal head	Dry or low to moderate exudate
Heel	Low to moderate exudate
Tip or top of toe	Pale granulation tissue with ischemia or bright red, friable granulation tissue with infection

A closer look at diabetic foot ulcers

This photo shows a diabetic foot ulcer on the plantar surface of the fifth metatarsal head. The circular shape of the wound is consistent with a wound created by pressure over a bony prominence.

This photo shows a pressure ulcer that has developed over the heel from impaired protective sensation and poor mobility.

This photo shows a pressure wound on the right lateral malleolus. Note the characteristic tissue changes associated with arterial insufficiency: thin, shiny skin; pallor; and muscular atrophy in the lower extremity.

Also note the calloused edges of the wound.

Ulcerations appear at the first and fifth metatarsal heads on this foot affected by Charcot's disease. Note the rocker bottom deformity.

Diabetic foot ulcers typically occur at sites of pressure, as in this heel ulcer.

Classification

Classifying diabetic ulcers helps ensure that all members of the health care team provide treatment appropriate to the ulcer's severity.

Depending on the classification system, diabetic foot ulcers are classified according to depth, presence of ischemia, and presence of infection.

University of Texas Diabetic Foot Classification System

The University of Texas Diabetic Foot Classification System provides a detailed categorization, which includes infection and ischemia.

Stage	Grade 0	Grade I	Grade II	Grade III
A	Preulcerative or post-ulcerative foot at risk for further ulceration	Superficial ulcer without tendon, capsule, or bone involvement	Ulcer penetrating to tendon or joint capsule	Ulcer penetrating to bone
B	Presence of infection	Presence of infection	Presence of infection	Presence of infection
C	Presence of ischemia	Presence of ischemia	Presence of ischemia	Presence of ischemia
D	Presence of infection and ischemia	Presence of infection and ischemia	Presence of infection and ischemia	Presence of infection and ischemia

This isn't like in school. In this instance, a low score is a good thing.

Wagner Ulcer Grade Classification

In the Wagner Ulcer Grade Classification, less-complex ulcers receive lower scores; more-complex ulcers, higher scores. Ulcers with higher scores may require surgical intervention or amputation.

Grade	Characteristics
0	■ Preulcerous lesion ■ Healed ulcer ■ Presence of bony deformity
1	■ Superficial ulcer without subcutaneous tissue involvement
2	■ Penetration through the subcutaneous tissue; may expose bone, tendon, ligament, or joint capsule
3	■ Osteitis, abscess, or osteomyelitis
4	■ Gangrene of a digit
5	■ Gangrene requiring foot amputation

Treatment

Successful ulcer healing depends on proper wound care and off-loading. The care plan may also include debridement, antimicrobials, biotherapies, and surgery.

Treatment algorithm for diabetic ulcers

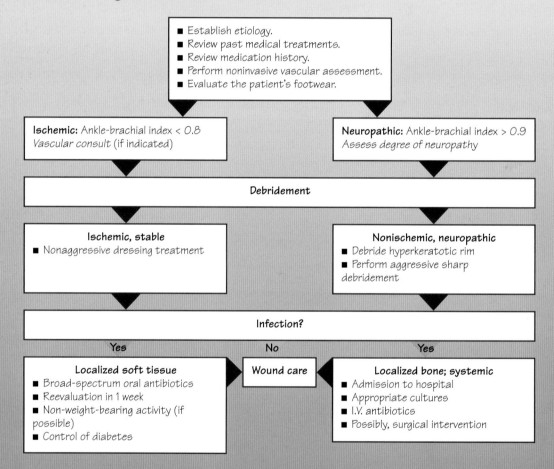

- Establish etiology.
- Review past medical treatments.
- Review medication history.
- Perform noninvasive vascular assessment.
- Evaluate the patient's footwear.

Ischemic: Ankle-brachial index < 0.8
Vascular consult (if indicated)

Neuropathic: Ankle-brachial index > 0.9
Assess degree of neuropathy

Debridement

Ischemic, stable
- Nonaggressive dressing treatment

Nonischemic, neuropathic
- Debride hyperkeratotic rim
- Perform aggressive sharp debridement

Infection?

Yes   No   Yes

Localized soft tissue
- Broad-spectrum oral antibiotics
- Reevaluation in 1 week
- Non-weight-bearing activity (if possible)
- Control of diabetes

Wound care

Localized bone; systemic
- Admission to hospital
- Appropriate cultures
- I.V. antibiotics
- Possibly, surgical intervention

Wound care algorithm for diabetic ulcers

Evaluate patient.

Evaluate footwear.

Surgical referral for bony deformities

Wagner Grade 0	**Wagner Grade 1**	**Wagner Grade 2**	**Wagner Grade 3**	**Wagner Grades 4 and 5**
■ Padding and accommodative devices ■ Callus debridement	■ Follow Grade 0 protocol ■ Topical silver sulfa-diazine (Silvadene) on highly contaminated wounds ■ Nonocclusive dressing ■ Weekly evaluation until healed ■ Plantar surface—gauze dressing ■ Dorsal surface—occlusive or non-occlusive dressing ■ Growth factor (beca-plermin [Regranex]) when ankle-brachial index is > 0.45	■ Follow Grade 1 protocol ■ Rule out osteomyelitis (X-ray, bone scan, bone biopsy) ■ Non-weight-bearing activity ■ Surgical consult ■ Plantar surface—gauze, amorphous hydrogel, alginate, or foam dressing ■ Dorsal surface—occlusive dressing ■ Topical antimicrobial cream, ointment, or amor-phous hydrogel ■ Growth factor (becaplermin [Regranex]) when ankle-brachial index is > 0.45	■ Follow Grade 1 protocol ■ Rule out osteomyelitis (X-ray, bone scan, bone biopsy) ■ Plantar surface—gauze, amorphous hydrogel, alginate, or foam dressing ■ Dorsal sur-face—nonocclusive dressing ■ Topical anti-microbial cream, ointment, or amor-phous hydrogel	■ Surgical consult and intervention

Best dressed

Dressings for diabetic foot ulcers

Type of ulcer	Recommended dressings
Dry	■ Hydrogel
Wet	■ Alginate ■ Foam ■ Collagen
Shallow	■ Transparent film ■ Hydrocolloid
Tunneling or deep	■ Alginate ropes (for wet ulcers) ■ Hydrogel impregnated gauze (for dry ulcers)
Infected	■ Iodosorb (a gel that cleans the wound by absorbing fluid, exudate, and bacteria) ■ Acticoat or Arglaes (products with an antimicrobial component)
Bleeding	■ Alginate

Off-loading

Patients with diabetic neuropathy no longer feel the pain that normally precedes tissue damage. Therefore, relieving pressure from plantar tissues—known as *off-loading*—is key to treating and preventing ulcers. Off-loading can be accomplished using nonsurgical and surgical interventions.

Nonsurgical interventions

- Therapeutic footwear (possibly with rocker soles)

This shoe has a toe box with extra depth and width to accommodate bony deformities, such as claw toes and hallux valgus (displacement of the great toe toward other toes). The shoe can also be modified to allow room for a widened hindfoot. The soft, thick inlay provides comfort and protection.

- Custom orthotics
- Walking casts (such as a total contact cast)
- Walkers
- Splints

This ankle-foot orthosis is used to relieve pressure from the heel.

Surgical interventions

- Exostectomy
- Digital arthroplasty
- Bone and joint resections
- Partial calcanectomy

Keep in mind that using an off-loading device can increase the patient's risk of falling. Be sure to teach the patient about fall prevention.

Prevention

Comprehensive foot care programs can reduce ulcer-related amputation rates by up to 50%.

Diabetic ulcer prevention starts with teaching patients how to control diabetes and how to care for their feet.

Teaching topic	Teaching tips
Diabetes control	▪ Emphasize the importance of controlling diabetes. Discuss the consequences of failing to control diabetes (such as peripheral neuropathy and vascular damage). ▪ Explain that careful glycemic control can reduce the frequency and severity of neuropathy in people with type 1 or type 2 diabetes.
Foot hygiene	▪ Check feet daily for injury or pressure areas (using a long-handled mirror may make viewing easier). ▪ Wash feet with a mild soap, and dry thoroughly between the toes. ▪ Before getting in, check bath water to make sure it isn't too hot. (Test the water with an elbow, use a thermometer, or ask a family member to help). ▪ Apply a moisturizing cream to feet to prevent dry, cracked skin and to balance skin pH. Don't apply moisturizer between the toes. ▪ Cut toenails off squarely. Consult a podiatrist if toenails are deformed and thickened. ▪ Don't go barefooted; the risk of injury is too great.
Choosing socks	▪ Use silver ion–lined socks for fungus control, if needed. ▪ Wear white or light-colored socks to make bleeding from trauma easy to detect. ▪ Wear natural fiber socks (which breathe better than synthetics). ▪ Choose socks that wick perspiration away from the feet (such as cotton-blended socks) to prevent maceration. ▪ Use diabetic padded socks for shear and friction control.
Choosing shoes	▪ Wear shoes that fit well, not shoes that are too tight or loose. ▪ Wear shoes that breathe to reduce maceration and fungal infections. ▪ Wear new shoes for short periods (less than 1 hour) each day initially; gradually increase the time as your feet adjust. ▪ If you have any foot deformities or have a history of ulceration, wear professionally fitted shoes. ▪ If possible, wash your shoes to destroy microorganisms. ▪ Check your shoes before putting them on to make sure they don't contain anything that could cause an injury.

Show and tell

Describe the pathophysiology of sensory neuropathy illustrated here.

1. _____
   _____
   _____

2. _____
   _____
   _____

Able to label?

Identify the bony abnormalities associated with diabetic motor neuropathy on this illustration.

1. _____

2. _____

3. _____

9
Malignant wounds

Talk about a sad story! Malignant wounds set the stage for a number of challenges for both the patient and the caregiver.

Causes

Malignant wounds develop when a primary or metastatic tumor infiltrates the epidermis. Occurring in 6% to 10% of cancer patients, these wounds grow rapidly and commonly invade surrounding tissues and organs, creating sinus tracts and fistulas. Having a cauliflower-like appearance, malignant wounds are poorly perfused with friable, fragile blood vessels and contain large amounts of necrotic tissue.

Malignant wounds most commonly occur in patients with breast cancer. However, they may also occur in patients with cancer of the head, neck, chest, and abdomen as well as in those with leukemia, lymphoma, and melanoma.

Necrotic areas

Cancer cells

Sinus tract

Epidermis

Dermis

Subcutaneous tissue

Muscle

Fragile, friable blood vessels

Cancer cells invading surrounding tissue

◄ This squamous cell carcinoma, after being neglected, ulcerated to form the malignant wound shown here.

This basal cell carcinoma was also neglected. It eventually ulcerated and invaded deeper tissue. ▶

Malignant wounds can develop from a skin cancer that has been neglected.

◄ This photo shows an inflamed carcinoma of the breast.

The malignant wound shown here resulted when a lymphoma metastasized to the patient's scalp. ▶

When a primary tumor outgrows its blood supply, it can invade the skin, resulting in a malignant wound.

◄ This photo shows a squamous cell carcinoma arising from a burn scar.

Chronic wounds, or even scar tissue, may evolve into a malignant wound. This type of malignant wound is called a Marjolin's ulcer.

Complications

Problem	Causes	Management strategies
Odor	Nonviable, necrotic tissue and excessive drainage create an ideal environment for bacterial growth. In turn, this produces a foul odor. Odor-causing aerobic bacteria include Klebsiella, Proteus, Pseudomonas, and Staphylococcus. Anaerobic bacterial causes include Clostridium and *Bacteroides fragilis*.	• Change dressings and gently irrigate the wound with normal saline solution at frequent intervals. • Apply topical antibiotics to reduce the amount of bacteria. • Use other topical antimicrobials, such as metronidazole gel (MetroGel), crushed metronidazole tablets, or silver sulfadiazine (Silvadene), as indicated. • Use charcoal dressings, such as CarboFlex and Actisorb Plus. • Apply mentholatum (Vicks VapoRub) near the patient's or caregiver's nostrils to minimize the perception of odor. • Place a tray of kitty litter, baking soda, or charcoal under the patient's bed to absorb odors. • Apply a pouching system to the wound to help control odors.
Bleeding	Malignant cells secrete tissue permeability factor, which increases vascular permeability and promotes a loss of protein and fibrinogen. This causes the blood vessels surrounding a malignant wound to become friable and fragile, and the blood to have an impaired ability to clot.	• Use nonadherent dressings (such as silicone dressings) to minimize tissue trauma and reduce the risk of bleeding. • Avoid frequent or unnecessary dressing changes. • Apply sucralfate (Carafate) suspension or paste to the surface of friable blood vessels to provide barrier protection. • Assist with surgical intervention (cauterization) or the application of topical epinephrine (Adrenalin) 1:1000 to control profuse bleeding. • Apply silver nitrate sticks or topical thrombin (Thrombin-JMI) to control sudden, profuse bleeding. • Administer oral antifibrinolytics (such as tranexamic acid [Cyklokapron]), as prescribed, to control severe bleeding.
Exudate (drainage)	The leakage of fibrinogen and plasma colloids by vessels in the wound causes exudate to form. Bacteria in the wound release enzymes that liquefy tissue, producing additional exudate.	• Use highly absorbent dressings (such as calcium alginate, foam, and hydrofiber) in wounds with moderate to large amounts of exudate. • Administer topical or systemic antimicrobials, as prescribed, to reduce bacterial load and exudate. • Use a wound drainage system, such as a pouch, on wounds with large amounts of exudate. (Avoid using a negative pressure system.) • Protect the surrounding skin from maceration and irritation.
Pruritus (itching)	As malignant cells invade surrounding tissue, the skin stretches and the peripheral nerves become irritated, commonly resulting in pruritus. Fungal infections may also cause pruritus.	• Chill hydrogel sheet dressings in the refrigerator and then apply to the wound. • Apply menthol creams to the affected area. • Advise the patient to use cool or lukewarm water to bathe or shower, rather than hot water. • Tell the patient to use a cool mist humidifier during colder months. • Advise the patient that antihistamines typically have no effect on the pruritus associated with malignant wounds.
Pain	Pressure on nerve endings from the tumor as well as exposure of the dermis to air may cause chronic pain. Dressing changes and other procedures may also worsen pain.	• Use a reliable and valid pain assessment tool—such as the visual analog, numeric pain intensity, or FACES pain-rating scales—to accurately assess the patient's level of pain. • Administer prescribed pain medication or topical anesthetics as ordered and before changing dressings or performing procedures.

Treatment

The goal behind any wound management system is to protect the wound and the surrounding areas and to provide an ideal environment for healing. However, because malignant wounds tend to occur near the end of a patient's life, treatment typically focuses on controlling symptoms rather than on healing.

Best dressed

Dressings used for malignant wounds

Wound characteristics	Dressings	Medications
Exudate	• Foam • Calcium alginates • Hydrofibers • Mesalt	• Antibiotic creams
Odor	• Foam • Calcium alginates • Hydrofibers • Composite • Charcoal • Occlusive	• Topical metronidazole • Antibiotic creams
Pain	• Hydrogels (if wound has minimal drainage) • Foam • Calcium alginates • Hydrofibers • Nonadhesive	• Topical anesthetics • Oral or parenteral pain medications
Bleeding	• Foam • Hydrofibers • Hemostatic (such as Gelfoam, Spongostan, and Oxycel)	• Topical epinephrine (use with caution) • Silver nitrate (to cauterize bleeding)

Because it's easier to control drainage, odor, and bleeding in a small wound, chemotherapy and radiation treatments are sometimes used to reduce the size of a malignant wound.

Matchmaker

Match the five complications of malignant wounds shown on the left with the management strategies shown on the right.

1. Odor _____
2. Bleeding _____
3. Exudate _____
4. Pruritus _____
5. Pain _____

A. Administer analgesics as ordered.
B. Use nonadherent dressings.
C. Apply topical antimicrobials to the wound.
D. Use a wound drainage system such as a pouch.
E. Apply cooled hydrogel sheets to the wound.

Rebus riddle

Sound out each group of symbols and letters to reveal the disease most likely to give rise to a malignant wound.

10

Wound care products

A dressing is to a wound like a costume is to a character. The right one makes all the difference.

Development of wound care products

Over time, wound care has evolved from a fairly rudimentary practice that focused primarily on the injury to a process that takes the patient's overall health into account.

Dressings

Selecting the right dressing for a wound means taking into account:
- the size of the wound
- the amount of moisture in the wound
- whether the wound is infected
- the condition of the surrounding skin.

> Controlling the amount of moisture in a wound is crucial to the healing process. That's why dressings are commonly classified according to whether they add moisture to a wound bed or whether they absorb it.

Dressing moisture scale

Use this chart to quickly determine the category of dressing that's appropriate for your patient.

Absorb moisture		Neutral (maintain existing moisture level)		Add moisture	
Alginates	Foams	Composites	Transparent films	Sheet hydrogels	Amorphous hydrogels
Specialty absorptives	Hydrocolloids		Biologicals		
Gauze	Wound fillers		Collagen dressings		
			Contact layers		

> This iodine-treated gauze is the greatest thing since sliced bread.

> Um, sliced bread hasn't been invented yet.

> Hmm…This patient is malnourished and has diabetes. That will definitely influence how I treat this wound.

> Keep in mind that new wound care products are being developed all the time, while old products are being improved. Make sure you stay up-to-date on all the "new releases."

The BIJOU
COMING ATTRACTIONS
COMING ATTRACTIONS

Alginate dressings

Made from seaweed, alginate dressings are available as sterile pads, ribbons, or ropes. These nonocclusive dressings are nonadherent and promote autolytic debridement to soften and remove necrotic tissue.

Alginate dressing in rope form

Very soft, nonwoven fibers turn into a biodegradable gel as they absorb exudate.

Fibers encourage hemostasis in minimally bleeding wounds.

And now, I'm proud to introduce the cast of characters in our wound care epic. In alphabetical order—beginning with alginate dressings and ending with wound fillers—let's hear it for the dressings of today!

To facilitate dressing removal—and to make dressing changes less painful—saturate the dressing with normal saline solution before removal. Use additional saline to clean the wound of any remaining dressing fibers.

Antimicrobial dressings

Antimicrobial dressings contain ingredients such as silver, iodine, and polyhexethylene to protect against bacteria. Available in various forms—including transparent dressings, gauze, island dressings, foams, and absorptive fillers—some antimicrobial dressings also provide a moist environment for wound healing.

> Besides making beautiful jewelry, silver has powerful antimicrobial and bactericidal properties. In fact, it's been used for centuries to prevent and treat infection.

> Silver in the dressing attacks bacteria and helps bind toxins.

Silver-impregnated antimicrobial dressing

Silver-impregnated activated charcoal cloth

Silver ions

Bacteria

Bacteria leaking fluid as it dies

How antimicrobial dressings work

Signs of wound infection include redness, swelling, and increased pain. If that isn't bad enough, infection can stop the healing process and worsen wound breakdown.

Once applied, an antimicrobial dressing immediately begins to release silver in a controlled fashion. The silver destroys bacteria in the dressing and the wound. Many antimicrobial dressings also absorb drainage and help keep the wound moist for optimum healing.

Collagen dressings

Made with bovine or avian collagen, collagen dressings are available in sheets, pads, particles, and gels.

Collagen dressings encourage wound healing by stimulating the deposit of collagen fibers necessary for the growth of tissue and blood vessels.

These highly absorbent dressings also maintain a moist wound environment.

Make sure wound infection has been treated and necrotic tissue debrided before using a collagen dressing.

Collagen in particle form

Some bovine collagen is processed into fine particles, as shown here. These particles can then be shaken into a wound bed.

Mixing with moist exudate in the wound, the particles gel as they absorb many times their weight in excess fluid.

Composite dressings

Composite dressings combine two or
more types of dressings into one.
Typical layers include:

1 Waterproof,
vapor-permeable
film

2 Absorbent
foam layer

3 Silicone
inner layer

> By combining two or more materials into one
> dressing, composite dressings reduce confusion
> and make dressing changes a snap.

A closer look at a composite dressing

This composite dressing stimulates autolytic debridement while controlling
moisture.

A thin, transparent, semipermeable
film allows the exchange of gas and
water vapor while blocking bacteria.

A highly absorbent foam-type matrix
slowly releases ingredients that clean
and moisturize the wound.

The adhesive backing consists of a
breathable cloth.

Contact layer dressings

Made of woven or perforated material, contact layer dressings are single-layer dressings designed to lie directly on the wound's surface. A secondary dressing is then placed on top of the contact layer.

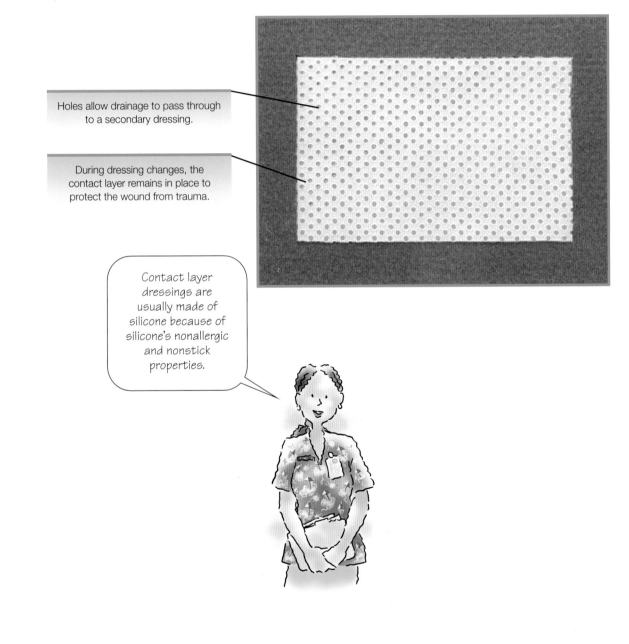

Holes allow drainage to pass through to a secondary dressing.

During dressing changes, the contact layer remains in place to protect the wound from trauma.

Contact layer dressings are usually made of silicone because of silicone's nonallergic and nonstick properties.

Foam dressings

Foam dressings are absorbent, spongelike polymer dressings. In addition to providing thermal insulation, they help create a moist wound environment.

Foam outer layer

- Provides comfort
- Allows water to evaporate
- Permits the free flow of oxygen and other gases

Inner contact layer

- Wicks drainage away from wound
- Allows trauma-free removal because of low adherence to wound surface

Adhesive foam dressing

This foam dressing has an adhesive border to secure the dressing over the wound bed.

Adhesive border   Nonadhesive contact layer   Foam

Nonadhesive foam dressing

This nonadhesive foam dressing has been cut to clearly show two distinct layers.

Nonadhesive contact layer   Top layer of semipermeable film

Hydrocolloid dressings

Made of a carbohydrate-based material, hydrocolloid dressings are adhesive, moldable wafers that are impermeable to oxygen, water, and water vapor. Besides being somewhat absorbent, these dressings help maintain a moist wound environment and promote autolytic debridement. These dressings are available in various thicknesses.

Hydrocolloids turn to gel as they absorb moisture, making the dressing become spongy and lighter in color over the wound. Reassure the patient that this is normal and, by itself, doesn't necessitate a dressing change.

Hydrocolloid dressing

This dressing, which is 2 mm thick, would be used on partial- and full-thickness wounds with exudate.

The exterior surface protects the wound from outside contaminants.

The hydrocolloid layer turns to gel as hydrocolloids absorb moisture.

The adhesive layer adheres to the surrounding skin, but not the wound; adherence decreases as gel forms.

Thin hydrocolloid dressing

Thin hydrocolloid dressings are used on superficial wounds with minimal exudate and to protect areas at risk for skin breakdown.

The hydrocolloid interior of this dressing is less than 1 mm thick.

Hydrocolloid paste and gel

Hydrocolloids are also available in paste, powder, and gel forms. Pastes and gels require a secondary dressing, such as a hydrocolloid wafer.

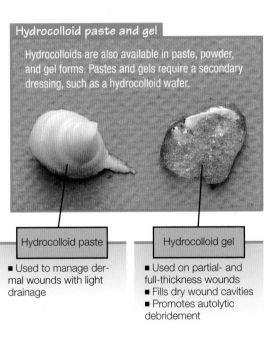

Hydrocolloid paste

- Used to manage dermal wounds with light drainage

Hydrocolloid gel

- Used on partial- and full-thickness wounds
- Fills dry wound cavities
- Promotes autolytic debridement

Hydrogel dressings

Made with a water or glycerin base, hydrogel dressings hydrate wounds and soften necrotic tissue. Because they contain a large percentage of water, these dressings provide limited absorption. Hydrogel dressings are available as a flexible sheet or a gel.

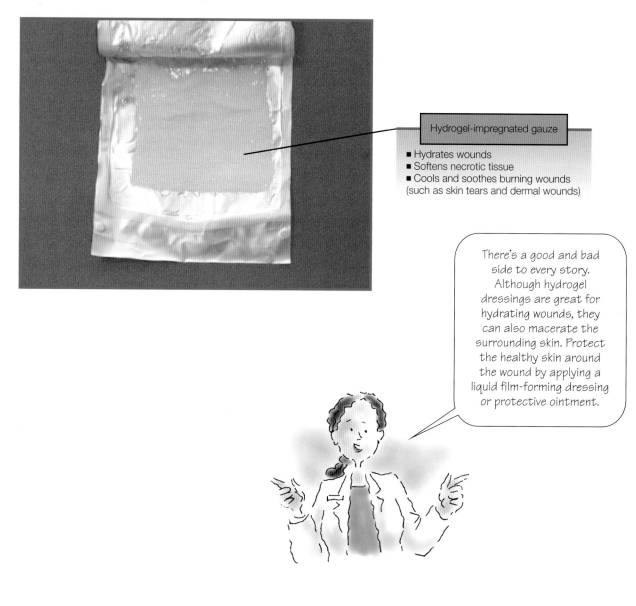

Hydrogel-impregnated gauze

- Hydrates wounds
- Softens necrotic tissue
- Cools and soothes burning wounds
(such as skin tears and dermal wounds)

There's a good and bad side to every story. Although hydrogel dressings are great for hydrating wounds, they can also macerate the surrounding skin. Protect the healthy skin around the wound by applying a liquid film-forming dressing or protective ointment.

Amorphous hydrogels

Amorphous hydrogels are gels packaged in tubes. Depending on the components in the gel, amorphous hydrogels have a number of uses.

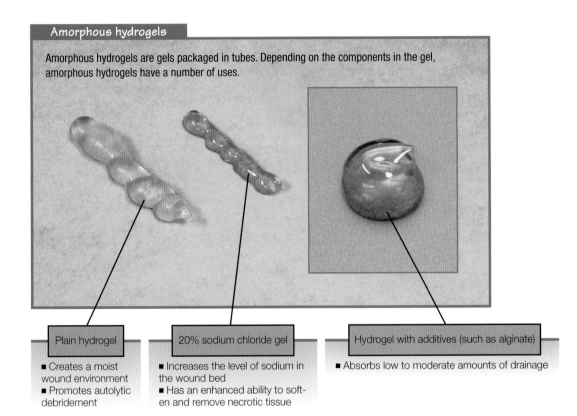

Plain hydrogel

- Creates a moist wound environment
- Promotes autolytic debridement

20% sodium chloride gel

- Increases the level of sodium in the wound bed
- Has an enhanced ability to soften and remove necrotic tissue

Hydrogel with additives (such as alginate)

- Absorbs low to moderate amounts of drainage

Specialty absorptive dressings

Specialty absorptive dressings, some with adhesive borders, contain multiple layers of a highly absorbent material, such as cotton or rayon. They're available as gels, pads, gauze, and pillows.

The abdominal pad is a mainstay for surgical wounds.

Thick cotton or polyfiber filling absorbs drainage well.

Soft woven cloth won't adhere to the wound bed.

Transparent film dressings

Made of polyurethane, transparent film dressings adhere to the skin and help maintain a moist wound environment. While these dressings are nonabsorbent, they promote autolytic debridement and stimulate the formation of granulation tissue.

Backing is removed before application, leaving a clear, membranelike dressing.

Film allows the exchange of water vapor and oxygen while being impermeable to fluids and bacteria.

Transparent film allows visual inspection of the wound while the dressing is in place.

Wound fillers

Used to fill deep wounds, some wound fillers add moisture to the wound bed whereas others absorb drainage. Made of various materials, wound fillers are available as pastes, granules, strands, powders, beads, and gels.

Wound filler in strand form

- Highly absorbent properties make it appropriate for wounds with heavy exudate.
- Strand form allows material to completely fill dead space.
- This particular filler contains silver, which has antimicrobial properties.

Wound filler in gel form

- Gel fills the wound evenly, helping prevent wound dehydration.
- Some gels effectively control wound odor.
- This dextrose-based gel mixes with wound drainage to coat and protect the wound and to provide a moist healing environment.

Wound care dressing review

Use this chart to quickly compare the various dressings, their indications for use, their advantages, and their disadvantages.

Dressing type	Indications for use	Advantages	Disadvantages
Alginates (Used as a primary dressing)	▪ Wounds with moderate to heavy drainage ▪ Wounds with tunneling	▪ Hold up to 20 times their weight in fluid ▪ May be cut to fit wound dimensions ▪ May be layered for more absorption ▪ Supplied in ropes for deep wound packing ▪ Promote autolytic debridement	▪ May require irrigation for removal ▪ Require secondary dressings ▪ Can't be used on dry eschar or wounds with light drainage ▪ May dehydrate dryer wounds
Antimicrobials (Used as a primary or secondary dressing)	▪ Infected wounds ▪ Wounds with minimal to heavy drainage ▪ Nonhealing wounds	▪ Help prevent or reduce infection ▪ Effective against a broad spectrum of microorganisms	▪ May produce a hypersensitivity reaction in patients sensitive to silver or iodine ▪ May sting when applied ▪ May contribute to the development of resistant organisms (not yet known)
Biologicals (Used as a primary dressing)	▪ Ulcers (specific product used will vary according to ulcer thickness) ▪ Skin graft donor sites ▪ Burns	▪ Promote healing ▪ Prevent infection and fluid loss ▪ Ease discomfort	▪ May cause allergic reactions ▪ May require secondary dressings
Collagens (Used as a primary dressing)	▪ Chronic, granulated wounds ▪ Wounds with tunneling ▪ Wounds with minimal to heavy drainage (depending upon specific product used)	▪ Available in various forms (gel, granules, and sheets; some also contain alginate) ▪ Perform well on chronic, clean wounds ▪ Conform well to wound bed ▪ Are nonadherent	▪ May cause an allergic reaction in patients sensitive to collagen, bovine, or avian products ▪ Require secondary dressings ▪ Aren't appropriate for third-degree burns or wounds with dry beds

(continued)

Wound care dressing review *(continued)*

Dressing type	Indications for use	Advantages	Disadvantages
Composites (Used as a primary or secondary dressing)	• Wounds with minimal to heavy drainage • Partial- to full-thickness wounds • Wounds with granulation tissue, necrotic tissue, or both	• Available in various combinations, sizes, and shapes • Conform well to wound bed • Promote autolytic debridement	• May not provide a moist wound environment (depending on the product selected) and may dry the wound bed • Can't be cut to fit without losing some dressing integrity • Can't be used on third-degree burns • Due to adhesive border, use may be limited if skin surrounding wound is fragile or nonintact
Contact layers (Used as a primary dressing)	• Partial- to full-thickness wounds • Wounds with minimal to heavy drainage • Skin graft donor sites	• Promote drainage to a secondary dressing while preventing the secondary dressing from adhering to the wound • Minimize pain during dressing changes • May be used with topical medications, fillers, or gauze dressings • Can be cut to fit or overlap the wound's edges	• Require a secondary dressing • Can't be used on stage I pressure ulcers, third-degree burns, infected wounds, and wounds with tunneling
Foams (Used as a primary or secondary dressing)	• Partial- to full-thickness wounds • Wounds with minimal to heavy drainage (including around tubes)	• Nonadherent • May be used alone (with an adhesive border) • Can be used on infected wounds if changed daily • May be used in combination with other products • Wick moisture from the wound and allow evaporation (hydropolymer foam dressings)	• Without an adhesive border, may require a secondary dressing, tape, wrap, or net • Aren't recommended for nondraining wounds • May cause maceration of skin surrounding wound if not changed regularly

Dressing type	Indications for use	Advantages	Disadvantages
Hydrocolloids (Used as a primary or secondary dressing)	▪ Partial- to full-thickness wounds ▪ Wounds with minimal to moderate drainage ▪ Wounds with necrosis or slough	▪ Nonadherent to a moist wound base ▪ Conform easily to the wound bed ▪ Maintain moisture by becoming gelatinous as they absorb drainage ▪ May be left in place up to 7 days, depending on wound characteristics ▪ Can easily be removed from the wound base ▪ Come in several forms and in both thin and traditional thicknesses ▪ Promote autolytic debridement ▪ Impermeable to water and bacteria	▪ May have an odor when removed ▪ Can't be used on burns or dry wounds ▪ Can cause skin stripping when removed ▪ Can cause maceration or hypergranulation ▪ May need to be held in place to maximize adhesion ▪ Aren't recommended for wounds with heavy drainage, sinus tracts, tunneling, or fragile periwound skin
Hydrogels (Gel or impregnated gauze forms are used as primary dressings; sheets are used as primary or secondary dressings)	▪ Partial- to full-thickness wounds ▪ Dry wounds ▪ Wounds with minimal drainage ▪ Wounds with necrosis or slough ▪ Infected wounds	▪ Available in sheet, strip, impregnated gauze, and amorphous gel forms ▪ Cool wounds to ease pain ▪ Add moisture to wounds ▪ Promote autolytic debridement ▪ Are easy to apply and remove ▪ Can be used to fill cavities or tunnels (gel or impregnated gauze forms)	▪ Require a secondary dressing (gel and impregnated gauze forms) ▪ Can macerate surrounding skin ▪ May necessitate daily dressing changes ▪ Not recommended for wounds with heavy drainage

(continued)

Wound care dressing review *(continued)*

Dressing type	Indications for use	Advantages	Disadvantages
Specialty absorptives (Used as a primary or secondary dressing)	• Infected or noninfected wounds with heavy drainage	• Are highly absorbent • Typically require less frequent changes • Are available in various forms • Are easy to apply and remove	• Can't be used on burns or on wounds with little or no drainage
Transparent films (Used as a primary or secondary dressing)	• Partial thickness wounds with minimal exudate • Wounds with eschar (to promote autolysis)	• May require less-frequent changes • Allow visualization of the wound • Aren't bulky • Are impermeable to bacteria	• Don't absorb drainage • Can strip the skin when removed; not for use on fragile skin • Can be difficult to handle and apply
Wound fillers (Used as a primary dressing)	• Infected and noninfected wounds • Wounds with minimal to moderate drainage • Wounds requiring packing	• Available in several forms with different capabilities • Can fill dead space in wounds • Are easy to apply and remove	• Require a secondary dressing • Can't be used on third-degree burns or dry wounds • Can alarm some patients because of the wormlike appearance of some products

Drugs and devices

Topical drugs and wound care devices can complement the function of dressings to promote wound healing.

To ensure that the debriding agent penetrates the tissue, crosshatch any eschar in the wound before application.

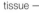 Debriding agents

Chemical or enzyme preparations called *debriding agents* are applied to necrotic or devitalized tissue to help facilitate its removal from a wound.

Necrotic tissue

1

First, apply the debriding agent to the surface of the wound.

2

Next, apply a dressing to seal in the debriding agent. The debriding agent then begins to digest and liquefy necrotic tissue.

3

Once or twice daily, remove the dressing and irrigate the wound to remove the liquefied necrotic material. Afterward, apply more debriding agent and a clean dressing.

Vacuum-assisted closure device

When a wound fails to heal in a timely manner, vacuum-assisted closure (VAC) may be used. The VAC therapy system consists of a special dressing, a vacuum tube, and a vacuum pump.

Region of subatmospheric pressure

Skin

Subcutaneous tissue

Muscle tissue

Bone

Wound base

Sealed dressing

Vacuum tube

1

One end of the vacuum tube is embedded in the foam dressing and the other connects to the vacuum pump.

2

When turned on, the pump gently reduces air pressure beneath the dressing, drawing off exudate and reducing edema in surrounding tissues. This process reduces bacterial colonization, promotes granulation tissue development, increases the rate of cell mitosis, and spurs the migration of epithelial cells within the wound.

Choosing a VAC dressing

The dressing used with a vacuum-assisted closure (VAC) device varies, depending upon the wound being treated.

> Choosing which dressing to use with VAC isn't always a black or white issue. For example, either dressing may be suitable for treating diabetic ulcers, dry wounds, skin grafts, shallow chronic wounds, and deep trauma wounds.

Black foam dressing

Benefits
The open, porous structure of this polyurethane dressing:
- stimulates the formation of granulation tissue
- evenly distributes negative pressure throughout the wound
- facilitates the removal of drainage.

Indications
- Deep acute wounds
- Deep pressure ulcers
- Flaps

White foam dressing

Benefits
This dense dressing made of a microporous polyvinyl alcohol material:
- reduces the growth of granulation tissue into the dressing (which reduces the pain of dressing changes)
- protects delicate structures
- prevents wound adherence.

Indications
- Wounds with sufficient granulation tissue
- Wounds with tunnels, sinus tracts, or areas of undermining
- Superficial wounds
- Painful wounds

Applying a VAC dressing

3

Apply the pad with tubing over the hole made in the drape.

2

Cut the drape to extend 1¼" to 2" (3 to 5 cm) over adjacent skin in all directions. Make a small hole in the center. Seal the drape securely.

1

Cut the foam dressing to fit the size and shape of the wound, extending it into areas of tunneling or undermining.

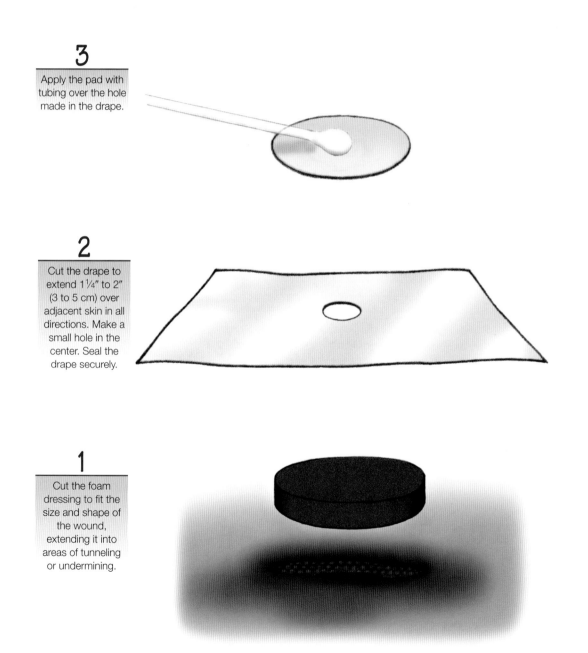

Provant wound-closure system

The Provant wound-closure system emits a radiofrequency signal into a wound to induce production of fibroblasts and epithelial cells and to trigger the secretion of multiple growth factors. This promotes wound healing, even in cases of chronic, severe pressure ulcers.

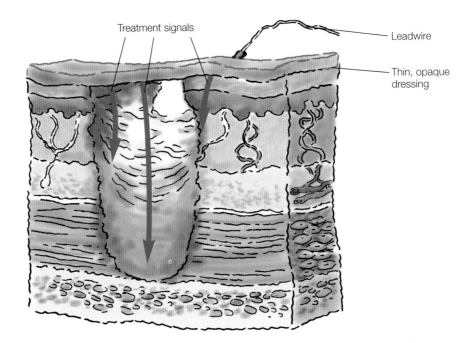

1

A treatment application pad (protected by a disposable cover) is placed over the wound. The dressing doesn't have to be removed.

2

The pad directs a radiofrequency signal 2¾" to 3¼" (7 to 8 cm) into the tissues around the wound. The signal triggers the:
- proliferation of fibroblasts, necessary for the development of granulation tissue
- proliferation of epithelial cells, necessary for wound closure
- secretion of multiple growth factors, to speed healing
- expression and activation of hundreds of genes controlling inflammation, granulation, epithelialization, and remodeling.

Treatment signals

Leadwire

Thin, opaque dressing

Warm-up therapy system

The Warm-up therapy system increases the temperature of the wound bed. This promotes healing by stimulating increased blood flow to the wound and by providing a moist wound environment.

1

First, a noncontact, raised foam ring with an adhesive border is applied to the wound site.

2

For wounds on distal extremities and toes, the foam ring is attached to a plastic sleeve.

3

A special electronic warming card is then inserted into the dressing. Once in place, the card heats to 100.4° F (38° C), bathing the wound in radiant, humidified heat.

Warming card

Review of wound care drugs and devices

Use this chart to quickly review the indications for use, advantages, and disadvantages of various wound care drugs and devices.

Drug or device	Indications for use	Advantages	Disadvantages
Debriding agents	▪ Wounds with moderate to large amounts of necrotic tissue ▪ Wounds in which surgical debridement is contraindicated	▪ May contain chlorophyll, which helps control odor ▪ Debride effectively even when used in small amounts	▪ May contain known allergens ▪ May require secondary dressings ▪ May irritate surrounding skin ▪ May cause a burning sensation in the wound that can last for several hours ▪ May turn drainage green (if product contains chlorophyll), leading to false concern of infection
Vacuum-assisted closure device	▪ Slow-healing acute, subacute, or chronic exudative wounds with cavities ▪ Pressure ulcers or surgical wounds more than 1 cm deep	▪ Cleans deeply and can manage moderate to large amounts of drainage ▪ Can manage multiple wounds when dressings are cut to bridge two or more wounds ▪ May allow patient mobility (some models have rechargeable batteries and are small enough to fit in a pouch worn at the waist or over the shoulder)	▪ Contraindicated for untreated osteomyelitis, malignancies, and wounds with necrotic tissue or fistulas ▪ Impairs mobility (vacuum tube is 5′ to 6′ [1.5 to 2 m] long) ▪ Requires electricity or rechargeable batteries to operate ▪ Can cause bruising at the wound base if the pressure is improperly set
Warm-up therapy system	▪ Acute or chronic, full- or partial-thickness wounds that have failed to heal with traditional therapies ▪ Wounds with compromised blood flow (such as arterial or diabetic foot ulcers)	▪ May absorb a small to moderate amount of drainage	▪ Contraindicated for third-degree burns ▪ Requires specific dressings and thorough patient teaching
Provant wound-closure system	▪ Wounds in the inflammatory phase of healing	▪ Requires no special training (patients can to perform therapy at home) ▪ Requires only two 30-minute treatments per day (device turns off automatically at the end of a session) ▪ May be used over existing dressings	▪ Contraindicated for use in pregnant patients and patients with cardiac pacemakers ▪ Won't promote healing of bone or deep internal organs

My word!

Use the clues to help you unscramble the names of three types of wound dressings. Then use the circled letters to answer the question posed.

Show and tell

Describe the steps for implementing warm-up therapy.

Question: Controlling the amount of moisture in a wound is crucial for what to occur?

1. These dressings contain multiple layers of highly absorbent material, such as cotton or rayon.

spaceylit vaporsbite

__ ◯ __ __ ◯ __ __   ◯ __ __ __ __ __ __ __

2. Made from seaweed, these dressings contain very soft, nonwoven fibers that turn into a biodegradable gel as they absorb exudate.

alientag __ __ ◯ __ ◯ __ __ __

3. These adhesive, moldable wafers are impermeable to oxygen, water, and water vapor.

coldhydrooil ◯ __ __ __ __ __ __ __ __ __ ◯ __

Answer: __ __ __ __ __ __ __

1. _____
_____
_____
_____

2. _____
_____
_____
_____

3. _____
_____
_____

Answers: My word! 1. Specialty absorptive; 2. Alginate; 3. Hydrocolloid; Question: Healing;
Show and tell 1. Place the raised foam ring with adhesive border on the wound site.
2. For wounds on the distal extremities or toes, attach the foam ring to a plastic
sleeve. 3. Insert a special electronic warming card into the dressing.

Selected references

Ayello, E.A., et al. "Nursing 2005 Wound Care Survey Report," *Nursing2005* 35(6):36-45, June 2005.

Bechara, F.G., et al. "Shave Therapy for Chronic Venous Ulcers: A Guideline for Surgical Management and Postoperative Wound Care," *Plastic Surgical Nursing* 26(1):29-34, January-March 2006.

Brown, P., and Maloy, J.P. *Quick Reference to Wound Care*, 2nd ed. Sudbury, Mass.: Jones & Bartlett Pubs., Inc., 2005.

Cutting, K.F., and White, R.J. "Criteria for Identifying Wound Infection—Revisited," *Ostomy/Wound Management* 51(1):28-34, January 2005.

Hess, C.T. *Clinical Guide to Wound Care*, 5th ed. Philadelphia: Lippincott Williams & Wilkins, 2005.

Hess, C.T. "The Art of Skin and Wound Care Documentation," *Advances in Skin & Wound Care* 18(1):43-53, January-February 2005.

Marston, WA. "Risk Factors Associated with Healing Chronic Diabetic Foot Ulcers: The Importance of Hyperglycemia," *Ostomy/Wound Management* 52(3):26-32, March 2006.

Maylor, M.E. "Establishing Nurses' Preferences in Wound Assessment: A Concept Evaluation," *Journal of Clinical Nursing* 15(4):444-50, April 2006.

McIntosh, C.D., and Thomson, C.E. "Honey Dressing Versus Paraffin Tulle Gras Following Toenail Surgery," *Journal of Wound Care* 15(3):133-36, March 2006.

Mendez-Eastman, S. "Use Negative-Pressure Wound Therapy for Positive Results," *Nursing2005* 35(5):48-50, May 2005.

Molan, P.C. "The Evidence Supporting the Use of Honey as a Wound Dressing," *International Journal of Lower Extremity Wounds* 5(1):40-54, March 2006.

Phelps, J.R., et al. "A Case Study of Negative Pressure Wound Therapy to Manage Acute Necrotizing Fasciitis," *Ostomy/Wound Management* 52(3):54-59, March 2006.

Pieper, B. "Wound Management in Vulnerable Populations," *Rehabilitation Nursing* 30(3):100-105, May-June 2005.

Posthauer, M.E. "Hydration: Does It Play a Role in Wound Healing?" *Advances in Skin & Wound Care* 19(2):74-76, March 2006.

Salcido, R.S. "Using Our Senses in Wound Care," *Advances in Skin & Wound Care* 18(1):8-11, January-February 2005.

Sargent, R.L. "Management of Blisters in the Partial-Thickness Burn: An Integrative Research Review," *Journal of Burn Care & Research* 27(1): 66-81, January-February 2006.

Schuster, R., et al. "The Use of Vacuum-Assisted Closure Therapy for the Treatment of a Large Infected Facial Wound," *The American Surgeon* 72(2):129-31, February 2006.

Smith, S. "Successful Outcomes with the H.E.A.L. Program," *Ostomy/ Wound Management* 52(3):40-46, March 2006.

Sweitzer, S.M., et al. "What is the Future of Diabetic Wound Care?" *The Diabetes Educator* 32(2):197-210, March-April 2006.

Vlahakis, N.E. "Is Erythropoietin the Key to Optimize Wound Healing?" *Critical Care Medicine* 34(4):1279-80, April 2006.

Credits

Chapter 1

Epidermal layers, page 4. Premkumar, K. *The Massage Connection Anatomy and Physiology*. Baltimore: Lippincott Williams & Wilkins, 2004.

Blood supply, page 5. Rubin, E. & Farber, J.L. *Pathology*, 3rd ed. Philadelphia: Lippincott Williams & Wilkins, 1999.

Chapter 3

Stage III pressure ulcer, page 37. Reprinted with permission from the National Pressure Ulcer Advisory Panel slide series #1. Available: *www.npuap.org.*

Chapter 4

Cleaning a wound, pages 40-41; Packing a wound, page 45; Hydrocolloid dressing, page 48; Moist saline gauze, page 49, Lynn, P. *Taylor's Clinical Nursing Skills: A Nursing Process Approach*. Philadelphia: Lippincott Williams & Wilkins, 2007.

Nonviable tissue and healthy tissue, page 54. From Fleisher G.R., et al. *Atlas of Pediatric Emergency Medicine*. Philadelphia: Lippincott Williams & Wilkins, 2004.

Chapter 5

Sunburn, page 58; Superficial partial-thickness burn, page 60; Postoperative infection, page 71. Images provided by Stedman's.

Partial-thickness sunburn, page 60; Deep partial-thickness burns, page 61; Full-thickness burn, page 63 (top). From Fleisher G.R., et al. *Atlas of Pediatric Emergency Medicine*. Philadelphia: Lippincott Williams & Wilkins, 2004.

Third-degree hand and wrist burn, page 63 (middle); Third-degree foot burn, page 63 (bottom). © English, MD/Custom Medical Stock Photo.

Electrical burn, page 64 (bottom). Rubin, E. & Farber, J.L. *Pathology*, 3rd ed. Philadelphia: Lippincott Williams & Wilkins, 1999.

Types of skin grafts, page 68, and Common donor sites, page 69. Smeltzer, S.C. and Bare, B.G. *Brunner and Suddarth's Textbook of Medical-Surgical Nursing*, 10th ed. Philadelphia: Lippincott Williams & Wilkins, 2003.

Dermatome, page 69. © English, MD/Custom Medical Stock Photo.

Chapter 6

Braden scale, pages 86 and 87. Copyright 1988. Barbara Braden and Nancy Bergstrom. Reprinted with permission. All rights reserved. Permission to use this tool in clinical practice may be obtained, usually free of charge, at *www.bradenscale.com.*

Norton scale, page 88. Doreen Norton, Rhoda McLaren, and A.N. Exton-Smith, *An Investigation of Geriatric Nursing Problems in Hospital 8*. National Corporation for the Care of Old People (now Centre for Policy on Ageing), London, 1962.

Support surface characteristics, page 91; Management of pressure ulcers algorithm, page 99; Nutritional assessment and support algorithm, page 100; Management of tissue loads algorithm, page 101; Managing bacterial colonization and infection algorithm, page 102. *Source:* "Treatment of Pressure Ulcers." Clinical Practice Guideline Number 15, AHCPR Publication Number 95-0652: December 1994.

PUSH tool, page 94. Copyright National Pressure Ulcer Advisory Panel, 1998. Adapted with permission.

Deep tissue injury, page 95. Courtesy of Joyce M. Black, PhD, RN. Associate Professor, University of Nebraska Medical Center, College of Nursing.

Pressure ulcers, stages I to IV, pages 95–98. From Nettina, Sandra M., MSN, RN, CS, ANP. *The Lippincott Manual of Nursing Practice*, 7th ed. Lippincott Williams & Wilkins, 2001.

Chapter 7

Lymphatic system, page 112. Premkumar, K. *The Massage Connection Anatomy and Physiology.* Baltimore: Lippincott Williams & Wilkins, 2004.

Venous stasis ulcer, page 115 (left); Stasis dermatitis with venous ulcer, page 116 (top). Goodheart, H.P. *Goodheart's Photoguide of Common Skin Disorders*, 2nd ed. Philadelphia: Lippincott Williams & Wilkins, 2003.

Chronic venous ulcer, page 115 (right); Advanced chronic venous ulcer, page 116 (bottom); Arterial insufficiency, page 120 (left). Marks, R. *Skin Disease in Old Age.* Philadelphia: J.B. Lippincott, 1987.

Venous stasis ulcer, page 116 (middle). Weber, J., & Kelley, J. *Health Assessment in Nursing*, 2nd ed. Philadelphia: Lippincott Williams & Wilkins, 2003.

Arterial emboli ulcers, page 119; Gangrene, page 120 (right). Smeltzer, S.C. and Bare, B.G. *Brunner and Suddarth's Textbook of Medical-Surgical Nursing*, 10th ed. Philadelphia: Lippincott Williams & Wilkins, 2003.

Lymphedema, page 121. Rubin, E. & Farber, J.L. *Pathology*, 3rd ed. Philadelphia: Lippincott Williams & Wilkins, 1999.

Signs of lymphedema, page 122. Bickley, L.S. & Szilagyi,P. *Bates' Guide to Physical Examination and History Taking*, 8th ed. Philadelphia: Lippincott Williams & Wilkins, 2003.

Treatment of arterial ulcers algorithm, page 126. Adapted with permission from *Advances in Skin & Wound Care* 14(3):147, May-June 2001.

Chapter 8

Neuropathic ulcer, page 136 (left). Marks, R. *Skin Disease in Old Age.* Philadelphia: J.B. Lippincott, 1987.

Diabetic heel ulcer, page 136 (right). Goodheart, H.P. *Goodheart's Photoguide of Common Skin Disorders*, 2nd ed. Philadelphia: Lippincott Williams & Wilkins, 2003.

University of Texas Diabetic Foot Classification System, page 137. Adapted with permission from Armstrong, D.G., et al. "Treatment-based Classification System for Assessment and Care of Diabetic Feet," *JAPMA* 86(7):311-16, 1996.

Wagner Ulcer Grade Classification, page 137. Adapted with permission from Wagner, F.W., Jr. "The Diabetic Foot," *Orthopedics* 10:163-72, 1987. © Slack Incorporated.

Treatment algorithm for diabetic ulcers, page 138. Adapted with permission from *Advances in Skin & Wound Care* 13(1):35, January-February 2000. Wound care algorithm for diabetic ulcers, page 139. Adapted with permission from *Advances in Skin & Wound Care* 13(1):35, January-February 2000.

Chapter 9

Squamous cell carcinoma, pages 145 and 147. Goodheart, H.P. *Goodheart's Photoguide of Common Skin Disorders*, 2nd ed. Philadelphia: Lippincott Williams & Wilkins, 2003.

Basal cell carcinoma, page 145. Rubin, E. & Farber, J.L. *Pathology*, 3rd ed. Philadelphia: Lippincott Williams & Wilkins, 1999.

Inflamed carcinoma of breast, page 146. From Moore, K.L. & Agur, A. *Essential Clinical Anatomy*, 2nd ed. Philadelphia: Lippincott Williams & Wilkins, 2002.

Metastatic lymphoma, page 146. Image provided by Stedman's.

We gratefully acknowledge Anatomical Chart Company and LifeART for the use of selected images.

Index